Take Control Now

Your health is your responsibility

PAMELA CLARKE

◆ FriesenPress

Suite 300 - 990 Fort St
Victoria, BC, Canada, V8V 3K2
www.friesenpress.com

ISBN
978-1-4602-5834-7 (Hardcover)
978-1-4602-5835-4 (Paperback)
978-1-4602-5836-1 (eBook)

1. Health & Fitness, Naturopathy

Distributed to the trade by The Ingram Book Company

TABLE OF CONTENTS

ACKNOWLEDGEMENTS

My journey as a natural medicine practitioner began when my mother Averil Monica Smith (now deceased) introduced me to iridology in the early 1980s. My undying thanks to you, dear mother. Rest in peace.

To my wonderful family members, including my youngest daughter Alicia Clarke, who is an elementary school teacher (my little teacher) for her continuous encouragement throughout the process of writing this book.

And to my beautiful granddaughter Mikaela Clarke who patiently listened to my new ideas for this book.

I would also like to acknowledge my son Ajamu Clarke for all his technical support in formatting my typing and guiding me through all my computer difficulties. I am so proud to have a son like you. Thank you.

To my youngest son Reuben Dari, who is my creative advisor, I would like to thank you for your wise advice while I was writing this book. You took me out of my comfort zone and gave me a voice to speak about my encounter with cancer. Continue to motivate and guide your clients. Thank you.

And a special thanks to Alyssa Sun and Shaniqua Roberts for their assistance with technical support.

Thank you, Mr. Noel Farrell, for your brilliance in editing the first draft of this book.

Lastly, but most importantly, to my handsome husband Winston, thanks a million for your kind and patient support throughout the years. Your encouragement and motivation are greatly appreciated in writing this book. May the Almighty continue to bless you in all your future undertakings.

DISCLAIMER

This book is not a substitute for your doctor or pharmacist in any way. It is designed to offer historical uses of herbs, vitamins, and minerals. If you are sick, please contact your doctor or go to the nearest emergency department.

Neither the author nor the publisher assumes any responsibility if you prescribe any supplement for yourself.

PART 1

CANCER

The first part of this book will reflect my journey through the storm of cancer and how I took responsibility for my health during this crucial period of my life.

My first encounter with cancer was as a student nurse in Jamaica. I remember very clearly one of my patients, a young girl around the age of sixteen, had a malignant ovarian teratoma. This tumour contained a diversity of tissues such as nerves, hair, and teeth. I remember this young girl was gravely ill. She was treated with radioactive (60) cobalt therapy, but I'm sad to say she succumbed to the disease.

According to the *Encyclopaedia Britannica*, cancer is any one of a group of more than 100 related diseases characterized by the uncontrolled multiplication and disorganized growth of cells in the body. Our body is made up of cells. Each cell contains twenty-three pairs of chromosomes. Our chromosomes contain millions of different messages (genes) that tell the body how it should grow, function, and behave. These chromosomes reproduce themselves; every time a cell divides, there is a chance for abnormal growth.

A cancer cell continues to grow uncontrollably, eventually forming an outgrowth that is called a tumour (cancer). When the body is affected by disease, there is a change in its genetic code that makes it forget to stop growing. Once the growth is turned on, a cancer cell continues to divide in an uncontrolled way. Malignant (cancer) growth is aggressive and invades surrounding tissues, spreading to distant sites. It may eventually kill the host. Malignant tumours (cancer) have two characteristics:

Cancer cells grow like an unruly plant, without border. They will invade any surrounding tissues in their path.

When pieces of the malignant cells break away, they act like seeds floating in the wind and, wherever they land, they start a new growth.

WHAT CAUSES CANCER?

Sometimes I wonder if anyone knows the cause of cancer. Many researchers believe that certain things cause cancer, including the following:

- Environmental factors;
- Chemicals;
- Diet;
- Stress;
- Sexual and reproductive history;
- Heredity;
- Free radicals.

Recently, I heard some one on TV saying that some cancers could be caused by mere "bad luck."

I do not know anyone in my family who has had cancer, but I do not want to categorize my encounter with cancer as bad luck.

I will now examine what was happening in my life around the period when my body started to give me warning signals.

I had a part-time job working as a registered nurse at the hospital; during this period, I mainly worked weekend shifts.

I also worked part time in a pharmacy; I would work at the store when I had no classes scheduled.

I was enrolled in university as a full-time student.

I was responsible for the care of five children. The youngest of the children was eight years at the time, and they were all in school full time. I was responsible for preparing their meals, cleaning their clothes, and doing most of the housework.

I was not getting enough sleep. I remember many times studying for examinations I would start reading and, before completing one page, fall asleep.

I was not eating properly. I was very busy, so sometimes I would get fast food while on the go.

If I were looking at the above profile, I would assess the person in question as burning the candle at both ends and encourage her to evaluate what she was doing. I now see a very stressed woman who was trying to do too many things for too many people at the same time.

To put it bluntly, I was wearing too many hats, and I was playing with fire.

I remember one day I was speaking to one of my professors, and the topic came up about children and work. When I gave her a bird's-eye view of my life, she looked at me and bluntly said, "Who the hell do you think you are? You think you are superwoman? I have two children and find it hard to cope — what are you thinking?" I was taken aback by her comments because at that time I thought I was coping very well and following my dreams. In hindsight, I wonder if she could have been right.

What was I thinking and doing to my body?

STRESS AND DISEASE

Chronic stress can give rise to many physical illnesses such as digestive problems (ulcers), high blood pressure, infertility problems, and weakened immune systems. If your immune system is under constant stressful attack, it will gradually weaken, and illness and even malignancy can result.

LACK OF SLEEP

In my case, I was not sleeping very well. I would stay up studying until the wee hours of the morning and, on average, was getting just four to six hours of sleep. My body became accustomed to that amount of sleep, though, and I did not feel stressed. But I paid for it in a different way: I had high blood pressure.

EXAMINATION STRESS

Another form of stress I experienced came with studying and writing exams. In order to be successful, I had to make time to study. With five children — even though they were not babies — it was not that easy. As the day of my examination drew closer, I would often wonder if I was adequately prepared to write it.

WORK STRESS

There was also some work stress for me during this time, working the night shift on the weekend as I was. Sometimes, these shifts, which operated on reduced night staffs, would get very busy.

POOR DIET AND STRESS

During this period, my diet could be classified as culturally delicious, but lacking in most of the ingredients required for balance. Later in the paper, I will discuss my culturally palatable diet.

In hindsight, three critical factors could have contributed to the dysfunction of my immune system at this time in my life:

1. Stress.
2. Imbalanced diet.
3. Lack of exercise.

In early November 1994, I observed I was passing blood in my stool and, as a medical personnel, the first thing that came to my mind was cancer of the colon. However, immediately, I quieted my mind by saying, No way. There is not a family history of cancer. *I do not have cancer.*

I went to my family doctor and told him that I thought I had haemorrhoids and requested medication to treat them, which he prescribed. The medication/ointment did not resolve the problem. I think my doctor had the same suspicion I did because he made an appointment for me to see a surgeon who specialized in general and colon surgery.

I had a colonoscopy on December 3, 1994, and was diagnosed with colon cancer that same day. I could see the sadness in the surgeon's eyes when he said the results were positive for cancer. "I saw the tumour and would like to do surgery ASAP," he said. He wanted to know how I came to the hospital; I informed him that I came by myself. He insisted that I should not return home alone, so he called my husband who had to leave work to get me. Before I went home, blood was drawn for CEA, and an appointment was made for me to have surgery on December 7, 1994.

That evening when I went home, I decided not to tell the children the full details of my medical history. I wanted time to be by myself and away from the family. The only place I could think to go was shopping at the supermarket. I bought a lot of chicken and other groceries. That night I seasoned all the chicken, putting cooking portions in Ziploc bags. The family would have sufficient meat and food for an extended period.

The following Saturday morning, I received a call from the doctor. He asked, "Are you feeling exhausted?" I said I wasn't. He replied, "Your potassium level is very low and can be considered dangerous during surgery." He prescribed potassium bicarbonate tabs, with instructions to take one tab twice daily for three days.

I was admitted to the hospital on Monday, December 6, 1994. My potassium therapy was continued via intravenous therapy:

> 2/3 & 1/3 20 mEq KCL per 1L (20 mmol/L of potassium chloride in 3.3% dextrose and 0.3% sodium chloride). The solution was infusing at 75 drops per minute.

I had surgery the following morning.

The confirmed diagnosis was as follows:

> Carcinoma of the colon.

The operative procedure I had was as follows:

- Left hemicolectomy with anterior anastomosis (segmental resection).
- The diseased part of the colon, along with some healthy areas on both sides of the tumour, was also removed, as well as some nearby lymph nodes.

- The remaining healthy areas of the colon were attached (anastomosed).

Surgical pathology report:

- Adenocarcinoma of colon, moderately differentiated, extending through serosa.
- Resection margins — negative for malignancy.
- Metastatic adenocarcinoma in two of thirteen pericolonic lymph nodes identified.

SIGNS AND SYMPTOMS OF CANCER

Some of the signs and symptoms of cancer are as follows:

- Any noticeable changes in elimination habits (bowel and urinary).
- Slow-healing sores.
- Unusual discharges (blood).
- Growth or lump in the breast or other parts of the body.
- Problems swallowing or other digestive problems.
- Change in wart/mole.
- Uncontrollable coughing or hoarseness.

Cancer develops really slowly and is seldom found until obvious signs and symptoms are present. By this time, it is sometimes too late and, oftentimes, metastasis has already developed. As the disease progresses, pain, weakness, weight loss, and anemia are present. These symptoms do not appear until late in the disease process.

ENVIRONMENTAL FACTORS AFFECTING CANCER

Toxic environmental chemicals — pesticides and industrial waste — assault the body and poison the immune system.

CHEMICALS AND CANCER

- Smokers are at a significant risk of cancer of the lungs, throat, kidneys, mouth, bladder, and pancreas.
- Excessive consumption of alcohol has been linked to cancer of the mouth, larynx, throat, liver, breast, and esophagus.
- Estrogen replacement therapy (DES) prescribed for menopausal women increases the chance of cancer in the female organs and also the liver.
- Radiation can cause cancer of the lungs, breast, skin and throat, and also leukemia. This includes natural radiation from overexposure to the sun.
- Asbestos can cause cancer in the respiratory tract. This is a hazard to people working in shipping, mining, and construction.

DIET AND CANCER

Numerous researchers have shown that a very high percentage of cancers are linked to a high-fat and low-fibre diet. A high-fat diet dramatically increases the incidence of breast and colon cancer. For optimum cellular nourishment, proper nutrition is key.

During the years leading up to my cancer, my diet was based on the delicious foods of my Jamaican culture. Among them:

- escovitch fish (high-fat meat);
- curried goat ;
- deep-fried chicken (high-fat meat);

- fried plantain (high-fat food);
- coco bread (high in starch; made with white flour);
- bulla cake (high in starch and sugar);
- rice and peas (high in starch);
- fried dumplings (high in fat and starch);
- hard dough breads (high in starch);
- ackee and salt fish (the national dish of Jamaica; high in salt);
- salted mackerel (very high in salt);
- corned/bully beef (very high in salt);
- sweetened beverages (high in sugar);
- Jamaican patties (high in fat);
- Jamaican rum cake (high in sugar).

I am not saying that my diet had anything to do with my cancer. What I am saying and pointing to here is that, during that crucial period in my life, an analysis of the type of foods I was consuming reveals a diet that was neither very nutritious nor balanced. I was eating a lot of fat, starches, and sugar. My diet lacked fibre and included an insufficient amount of fruits and vegetables. However, I can say one thing about the foods I was eating then: they were appetizing. My taste buds are very cultural; I still love my Jamaican food. However, after my surgery, I stopped living by my taste buds; I am now living to survive. I am working with my body.

It now appears that my body has an inbuilt monitor, directing me to what foods I can eat. Where I could eat almost anything and suffer no problems whatsoever years ago, more recently, I have had to watch what I eat. If I put certain foods in my mouth, my body will shout at me: "Do not put that food in me!" Whenever I eat certain foods now, I will break out in hives, and my joints hurt very badly.

HEREDITY

It is believed that a familial tendency to cancer may exist and that individuals with such a history may be especially vulnerable to the disease. Bad genes can be transmitted from one generation to the next, allowing faulty genes in at a time (when the immune system is weakened) when they're needed to defend the body.

FREE RADICALS

Free radicals are the by-products or waste material expelled by cells, and they are normally not a threat to health. A problem arises, however, when too many free radicals are present in the bloodstream. This excess can circulate freely in the blood, damaging cells and overtaxing the immune system. Free radicals can do damage to DNA, causing cancer cells to multiply at a faster rate.

SEXUAL AND REPRODUCTIVE HISTORY

Many studies have been done on women whose many different sexual partners put them at risk for getting cancer of the cervix. This form of cancer is generally caused by HPV or human papillomavirus, and a woman can contract this viral infection by having a sexual encounter without using a condom, and by having many partners.

DIAGNOSIS

Sometimes, the symptoms are so typical that the diagnosis virtually proclaims itself. Other times, a doctor's suspicion is aroused by minor conditions not responding to treatment, an occurrence that warrants further investigatory tests. Self-tests are becoming very popular and have proven to be very important in helping with the diagnosis. These tests include the following:

- Breast cancer self-test: self-examination of the female breast is recommended as a safeguard against cancer of the breast. Early detection and prompt attention can save a woman's life.
- Colon cancer self-test: a test kit can be purchased at most pharmacies and used for detecting blood in the stool (an early sign of colon cancer). Blood found in the stool does not always signify cancer. Eating red meat or the presence of diverticulitis, haemorrhoids, polyps, ulcers, or an inflamed colon can cause blood to be in the stool. Only 10% of those with a positive test for blood in the stool have cancer.
- Testicular cancer test: After a warm shower or tub bath, use your fingers to check for nodules and lumps in the testes. This is a good practice.

Malignancy (cancer) in any area of the digestive system can remain undetected for a very long time, unless the individual is aware of the signs and symptoms that characterize malignancy in that part of the body. An annual check-up that includes a rectal examination with a proctoscope and a sigmoidoscope is beneficial for men.

A professional evaluation should be sought when the following symptoms are present:

- weight loss;
- anemia;
- poor appetite;
- any change in bowel habits such as: persistent constipation, diarrhea, or mucous or blood in the stool;
- cramps;
- rectal bleeding.

BIOPSY

By removing cells surgically or through aspiration for microscopic examination, a malignancy can be diagnosed.

CANCER SCREENING TEST FOR CEA

I have had this test done several times, and even though I am in the medical profession, just the thought of having a needle in my vein makes my whole body shiver. CEA is the short term for Carcinoembryonic Antigen. This procedure detects and measures a special protein that is not normally present in adults. CEA is secreted in the lining of the fetus's digestive tract during the first six months of fetal life. Normally, this antigen is not present at birth, but tumour growth can cause it to reappear in the blood later in life.

This test is used in the preoperative staging of colon and rectum cancers. It also sheds light on lung cancers, as well as some non-malignant liver, pancreas, and bowel disease.

MY DIRECT ENCOUNTER WITH CANCER

After completing my degree in psychology and graduating from York University in 1994, I was planning to study natural medicine at the Canadian College of Naturopathic Medicine. However, after learning that I had colon cancer, I felt that the tide had changed and I did not know how long I had to live. I felt that my dreams would not be actualized. I decided not to do any more studying. I wanted to spend the rest of my life dedicated to my children. I had radical surgery four days after the tumour was discovered. My surgeon stated that my CEA level was very high, so he wanted me to have the surgery ASAP.

HOW I OVERCAME CANCER

I was very fortunate to have a compassionate roommate. She was an elderly lady in her early seventies and had problems with a degenerative illness, which led to many hospitalizations. She was one of my sources of great support and strength. She was very comforting and always had words of encouragement for me.

Cancer is a critical and life-threatening condition, and as I lay on my sick bed, tears of agony and deep grief rolled down my cheeks day and night. I was thinking about my five young children. I cried, *What is going to happen to my children when I am gone?* I tried to pray, but I could only stare at the ceiling and the wall engulfed in deep sadness. Those tears were not for me; I knew that if I had died, I would be in a better place, and I would have no cares in this world. I would be gone, period.

One day I turned to my roommate, and told her I couldn't even pray. She replied, "What do you expect, when you are in the belly of the whale/ it's total darkness and you won't be able to pray." I pondered on her words *belly of the whale.* Then I remembered the story of Jonah in the Bible.

Jonah was commissioned to go and preach against the wickedness of the city of Nineveh by the Lord. However, he disobeyed, and went to Joppa and boarded a ship to Tarshish. While on the vessel, a great storm came upon the ship and threatened to sink it. Jonah told the crew that he was a disobedient Hebrew and was running away from the Lord, and said that if he was thrown into the rough waters, the storm would stop. Reluctantly, Jonah was thrown overboard and the storm stopped. While in the sea, Jonah was swallowed by a big whale, and he spent three days and three nights in its belly.

I pondered on the phrase "in the belly of the whale" and Jonah's time to think while mobilized in its belly. Jonah's experience transformed him into an obedient servant of God; he was strengthened and got the courage to carry out God's mandate to warn the people of Nineveh.

I started to think about what my "belly-of-the-whale" experience was going to mean. I then decided that to survive I would have to come out of the belly and fight for my life and those of my children. I love my children dearly and did not want another woman to raise them. I was not ready to call it quits, so I reached out to the greatest power on earth, **The Creator Of Heaven And Earth, The One Who Called Everything To Come From Nothing,** and I pleaded for a miracle.

I refused to die. I knew deep down within my being, within my soul, that I was going to live. I had to exercise my faith; I knew that I had to be strong. I gave God no other choice but to heal me, because I believed his words when he said in Matthew 11:28, "Come to me all you who are weary and burdened, and I will give you rest." I wanted rest and relief from my burden, from this illness, and I was going to trust my creator. My children mattered more to me than my pain; I placed them individually in my master's hand and prayed that he would give me more time with them. I trusted my God and I believe his words.

Death would have to take the back burner; death would have to wait. My job on this earth is not complete. I was put on this earth to support these children. I was blessed with them, and my work was not finished.

They would need me when the trials and tribulations of this life face them. I want to comfort them and help them. I know God is always in control, and he will never leave me helpless. Although I was fearful and scared, I knew deep within my heart that God would not forsake or leave me. So I silently telephoned heaven to my dear heavenly father.

I spent the next two weeks in hospital engaged in silent warfare.

I silently communicated with my best friend (Jesus), my forever friend who is still my daily companion and who has promised never to leave me.

For the duration of my stay in the hospital, I was very quiet externally; however, deep within my being, my telecommunication wire to glory was lit up. I was in a prayerful mood most of the time. **I knew that my prayers had touched heaven.** I imagined the angels saying, "Grant her wishes and give her more time with her children. Let it be, as stated in your words, my Lord."

I felt extremely weak. I remember saying to my surgeon, "Doctor, tell me something. When I came to the hospital I felt like I had normal strength, now I feel like I am one hundred years old." He did not give me an answer, but an understanding smile.

While in the hospital I was wrestling with whether to take chemotherapy treatment. My family doctor came to visit and encouraged me to take chemotherapy because my CEA level was extremely high prior to surgery.

A nursing educator and her students were on the unit, and they came to my room. The teacher also encouraged me to have the chemotherapy. Her sister-in-law had the same problem, she told me, and chemotherapy had helped her.

I was going through a very painful and dark time. It was one of the most painful days in my life. I felt like Daniel in the lion's den. I was in the valley of the shadow of death. However, I had faith. I knew deep within my being I was going to rise from my valley experience. I was going to see the light. I was going to have a brighter day.

I remember being in the recovery room after surgery and gaining consciousness. I have never had such excruciating pain, and after receiving the intramuscular injection, the feeling of dizziness that washed over my entire body was terrible.

I think that experience of being a patient made me into a better nurse. Even though I was always kind and understanding with my clients/patients, I was able to empathize more fully with them my after my experience.

If you have never had cancer, you will not have a clue what cancer sufferers have to endure. I have studied cancer; I have worked with cancer patients — both survivors and those that succumb to the disease. But even so, I was not fully prepared for what I had to endure. When you meet the *Big Bad C*, it is a different story. Let me briefly sum up my experience:

My feelings when I suspected that I might be a victim to that dreaded disease:

>At first, I was in denial. I did not believe this could be happening to me. To my knowledge, no one in my family has ever had cancer. Why me? I did not tell my family my fears because deep down inside me, I wished my problem would disappear.

My feelings when newly diagnosed:

>An overwhelming feeling of death and sadness overshadowed me.

>Many questions circulated in my mind.

>Who is going to take care of my children when I am gone? I know my husband is a responsible man, and that my children would be adequately taken care of. However, I don't think a man can replace a woman in child-rearing. My heart was completely broken for my five children.

>I was not at all thinking about myself. I know that when you are dead, you are dead. I would have no more pain, no

sorrow; I would just be gone off the face of the earth, leaving a grieving family behind.

I purposed in my heart:

I said to myself: I have to live, I am not ready to die — my children need me.

I prayed as I had never prayed before; my prayers went something like this:

My Dear Heavenly Father, the giver of all good things to mankind. You are the only real and true friend I have. You know me more than anyone else in this fallen world. You knew me before I was conceived in my mother's womb. You know my fears and my joys. I know you did not give me these children for me to leave them so early. Father, I put all my faith in you, and although my faith may be like a mustard seed, I know you will understand. Increase my faith. As you stated in your words, you are the healing "balm of Gilead," Genesis 37:25, "Come and touch me from the crown of my head to the sole of my feet. Take this infirmity from me and heal me. Your words clearly state that you were wounded for our transgressions, and bruised for our iniquities. And by your stripes we are healed. Lord, I know you have no hands but ours. Please use the hands of the surgeon to remove this illness from my body and heal me completely. I thank you for the breath of life that you have given me and will continue to give me. I know the doctors cannot give life, and their word is not final, but your everlasting word is. As I ask for your mercies, I pray for your supernatural healing and complete restoration to my body and spirit. These mercies I ask in the matchless name of your son, Jesus. Thank you.

17

I purposed within myself that I wanted to live.

I made a complete lifestyle change. This change did not happen immediately. I felt too weak and too sick to introduce all the health changes immediately. The changes that took place were shortly after my hospital release.

I changed my thought process.

I changed my diet.

I changed my sleeping habits.

After my release from the hospital, I had an appointment at the oncology department at Sunnybrook Medical Centre. This consultation was primarily for an opinion regarding adjuvant therapy. My surgeon clearly stated that he was most concerned for me in view of my very high CEA level. He continued in his letter to the oncologist, "This obviously is a poor prognostic factor. The ultrasound and CT scan after surgery did not show any evidence of metastatic disease, but I would be concerned that there may be occult disease there somewhere."

ADJUVANT THERAPY

This is the treatment given in addition to the primary or initial therapy that is often surgery. This additional treatment is used after a surgery that removed all detectable disease, but where there may be a risk of hidden disease left behind. Adjuvant therapy is in the form of chemotherapy, hormone therapy, or sometimes both.

My husband accompanied me on my first visit to the oncology department. Given that Sunnybrook was one of the leading teaching hospitals in Toronto, there were several doctors and health-care-professional trainees in the consultation room. I had taken an envelope with my medical and medication history from my oncologist surgeon to the medical oncologist and his team who would plan the course of my chemotherapy. During this consultation, the head of the oncology department stated that he wanted to start chemotherapy as soon as possible because my CEA levels before and after surgery were very high.

MY RESPONSE TO STARTING CHEMOTHERAPY

The head oncologist wanted me to start the chemotherapy the following Monday (my appointment was on a Friday). I took a very deep breath and asked the doctors in the room what they would do if they were in my position. Everyone in the room answered that they would take the treatment. Because I was so young, they reasoned, I stood a very good chance of beating the cancer.

However, I knew about the toxic effects of chemotherapy, which are…

- induced nausea and vomiting
- fatigue
- mouth sores
- neuropathy
- constipation
- diarrhea
- hair loss.

I looked helplessly in the eyes of the head oncologist and replied, **"My aversion to chemotherapy is if I take this (therapy) medication I *will* die."** He held my hand and stated, "Your CEA is very high — that is why we want to start the therapy. So go home and think very seriously about this major decision, and we will take it from there on Monday."

MY AVERSION TO CHEMOTHERAPY

Aversion is an intense dislike. Chemotherapy is the treatment of a chemical substance, mainly cytotoxic medications and other drugs for cancer and other diseases. Conventional medical science claims that chemotherapy has many health benefits.

That weekend was very hard for me. I was already feeling feeble and I knew how I would feel after the chemotherapy. So I decided I did not want to feel any worse after the chemotherapy. I would rather spend the remainder of my life with the little strength I had with my family than vomiting and being too weak to be of any good to myself or anyone else.

The following week I returned to the oncology department at Sunnybrook to give the oncologist my final decision about taking chemotherapy. I told him I would not be taking it, but added, "The only thing I fear is what might happen in the future, say two years down the road, if this thing returns again."

He held my hands and seriously looked into my eyes and said, "Do not think that way." That was the last meeting I had with the good oncologist.

MY LIFESTYLE CHANGE

I had done some iridology studies, so I understood a little about alternative medical treatments and detoxification. I decided I was going to turn over a new leaf in all aspects of my life, beginning with my diet. After a week of detoxification, using large doses of red clover tea with chaparral as my blood purifier, I adjusted my dietary regime as follows:

- three to four cups of red clover tea daily for three months (using two heaping tsp. of dried herbs in eight ounces of hot water, letting it steep for half an hour). This I took with no sugar or honey.

- No added sugar or honey.
- No red meat.
- No cow's milk (dairy products).
- Increase fruits and vegetables (during this period, I consumed so much carrots that my hands turned orange).
- No fast foods or processed foods.

PREVENTION TIPS AGAINST CANCER:

- Do not smoke or use chewing tobacco. Tobacco products have been directly linked to cancers of the lung, mouth, throat, pancreas, kidney, bladder, cervix, prostate, and colon.
- Stay out of the sun. Getting a tan is a sign of skin damage. Sunlight contains ultraviolet (UV) rays, which can lead to melanoma and other skin cancers, and contribute to premature aging. Use sunscreen outdoors to protect your skin from ultra-violent rays.
- Drink alcohol only in moderation. Excessive drinking can increase the risk of damaging the liver and digestive system.
- Exercise regularly to keep your body active.
- Get regular screening for cancer as part of your annual physical check-up.
- Men over 50 should ask their doctors about an annual PSA test.
- For women, an annual pap test can reveal if you have growths on the cervix and can reduce your risk for cervical cancer. If you are over 40, ask your doctor if you need regular breast screenings.
- If you were exposed to known carcinogens, be sure to follow all safety guidelines.
- Check if your home contains asbestos. It can lead to serious respiratory problems (cancer). Homes built before 1980 used asbestos.
- To limit exposure to carcinogenic chemicals at home, avoid aerosol cleaning products.

- Keep moving. Regular exercise can help you maintain a healthy body and reduce the risk of cancer. Increase your daily activity up to sixty minutes by walking, gardening, doing housework, and dancing.
- Know your family's medical history. If any close family members have been diagnosed with any form of cancer, inform your family doctor.

FOLLOW THESE DIETARY GUIDELINES:

- Eat lots of fruits and vegetables. Fruits and vegetables contain scores of chemicals believed to have cancer-fighting properties).
- Eat high-fibre foods. Whole-grain cereals, vegetables, and fruits that are high in fibre may help prevent colon cancer.
- Eat less cured meats. Foods like ham, bacon, bologna, and hot dogs contain nitrates that can make you more vulnerable to cancer.

It has now been over twenty years and all of my follow-up examinations, X-rays, CT scans, ultrasounds, and blood tests have been negative.

I returned to work at the Humber Regional Hospital on a part-time basis six months after I had my surgery. I decided that I would not tell any of my colleagues about my experience with cancer. I did not want anyone's sympathy. The group of ladies I worked with were very kind and considerate, and I know it would have been very difficult working with their kind of support. I imagined them giving me the easiest assignments and telling me to take breaks. I wanted to carry my full workload, to be a whole part of the team, and not be pitied or pampered. I seldom called in sick and I remember one day one of my colleagues said, "Pam is the healthiest one of us here. She does not eat any junk food like the rest of us." I smiled to myself and said inwardly, "little would you know."

Recently, I attended a funeral for a young girl who died of cancer. During the service, tears filled my eyes as I sat and listened to her family and friends testifying of her deep faith and devotion to our God, during her suffering and how he relieved her of her pain, and took her home to Heaven.

I could not help but wonder why the Lord saved me and not her. Then, I started thinking: My work on this earth is not yet complete. My children are now grown. I know my job is to continue helping the suffering of humanity. As long as my Lord and saviour give me life and strength, I will continue to practice humanitarian service.

I give thanks to my god everyday for his keeping strength and guidance. **To God be the glory and praise.**

PART 2

TAKING RESPONSIBILITY FOR YOUR HEALTH

INTRODUCTION

The second part of this book will highlight the importance of taking care of one's body, and the impacts the lack of care can inflict on the body and the mind if they're not properly taken care of.

One reason for writing a part two for this book is my dear mother. If she had taken more responsibility for her own health, I believe she would still be here with me, on this side of Jordan. Mom passed away in November 1997. She would have turned seventy-one in December of that year. Although she was a registered nurse, she did not get enough rest and did not pay enough attention to her own health. She was busy helping others (which was very good and rewarding), while her health was slipping, and she was not fully aware of it.

She did not reveal to the family that she had a problem with her blood sugar until it was far too late. Several months after she was officially diagnosed with diabetes, she stated that when she came to Canada her family doctor told her that her blood sugar was high, but she did not pay any attention to that warning. She did not take responsibility for her health; neither did her family doctor and it cost her life. To see such a vibrant, brilliant lady suffer so much was heart-rending. I am trying to prevent others from going down the same road.

I vowed in my heart that I am always going to "take responsibility for my own health," and whenever my body gives me warning signals, I will always take heed. I hope my bird's eye view into taking responsibility for your own health will help someone.

Your body is a house/temple in which your spirit/soul dwells. It is comparable to a car. You cannot drive a car without gas. Likewise, your body will not work properly or for very long without proper care. Oftentimes, we spend lots of time and money to repair our homes and cars, we go to the hairdresser, we do our nails — yet we often neglect our bodies.

This part of the book is intended to give you a *brief* overview of the different functions of your body's system, what they need to work efficiently, and what may happen if you do not take proper care of it. In other words, it is a **manual for your body** (like a manual for a car). If you know the functions of your body's parts, you should also know the potential problems that could arise if they're not properly taken care of.

Let it be known that it is your responsibility to take care of your body, and that your body will take care of your life. I have also researched ways of caring for our body/house/temple in a holistic way — helping to maintain the body in a state of health that will naturally fend off diseases: mentally, emotionally, spiritually, and physically — covering as many systems as possible. Bernard Jensen stated, "The true healing art is one in which we teach the patient to change living habits, to conform to natural laws so that, instead of having to rebuild a sick body, one can prevent disease in the first place."

TAKING RESPONSIBILITY FOR YOUR OWN HEALTH

"The body is alkaline by design, but acidic by function."
— Albert Szent-Gyorgyi

Good health should be a natural state for all human beings. Unfortunately, the majority of people don't know what good health is.

When I think about health, I think of a body free of diseases and any form of injury. This concept also includes mental stability and social adjustment.

When you were a child, you were cared for by your parents and other adults. Now as an adult yourself, you are totally responsible for your own health. No one else is. It is your body, and no one knows your body like you do. So why should you rely on anyone to take care of you? We are given one body in this life. We should love it, pamper it, respect it, care for it. Your body is a precious gift. Treat it with care, respect, and dignity. Care for your body the way you would care for someone you really love, like your child.

Where there is health, disease has to flee, and in this state, the mind is stable. Wellness refers to the state of living a healthy lifestyle. Therefore, I would say that health and wellness incorporate the whole picture of health. **Taking responsibility for your own health** is viewed as the pursuit of **wellness.** "The question of health and disease often comes down to individual responsibility. This responsibility means choosing a healthful alternative over a less healthful one. To achieve and maintain this health, you will need to focus on the "four cornerstones of good health."

These are:

- A positive mental attitude.
- A healthful lifestyle: exercise, sleep, and healthy habits.
- A health-promoting diet.
- Supplementary measures.

In order to be able to take responsibility for your health, you should have at least a bird's eye view of what constitutes your body/house and how each part works. It is very interesting that we know how our cars, boats, and vacuum cleaners work, but many of us have no clue how our bodies work. Putting it mildly, in order to be able to care for your body and take responsibility for your health, you should know how your body works. Your body is like a very **complex machine**. I like to call my body "**my chemical factory,**" and this body has many parts that work by themselves or in conjunction with others to carry our specific functions.

CHAPTER ONE

MY DREAM

After completing my post-graduate studies in naturopathy, I wanted to share some of the valuable health information I learned over the years with my clients and friends. I will be sharing a modified version of my thesis, "Taking responsibility for your own health," in this book — but before I begin, I will tell you how it all started.

As a young girl growing up in Jamaica, my dream was always to be a nurse, like my mother, to help suffering humanity.

My mother left me at a very young age to study nursing in England. Whenever I went to the hospital to visit sick friends or relatives, I would always see the nurses smartly dressed in their white uniforms hustling and bustling on the wards, and I would think of my mother or of myself in the future as a nurse.

When I was old enough to correspond with my mother, I was jubilant to tell her of my desire to be a nurse, just like her. Unfortunately, she did not share my enthusiasm. She wrote back to say that nursing is a noble and humanitarian profession helping the sick, but that it is hard work and entails some duties that are not too pleasant. She suggested I think about being a schoolteacher, also a noble profession, and one that nurtures the minds of the young and helps them to be decent, hardworking citizens of the world.

I was not too happy with that advice. I had made up my mind to be a nurse and help suffering humanity.

I've always enjoyed helping people, especially if they've needed genuine help. Back in Jamaica, I always heard older ladies talking about getting a wash out to help biliousness. I did not understand what that meant at the time; however, as I got older and wiser, I understood that they meant detoxing or cleansing the liver, to help strengthen the body and build the body's immune system. I heard them saying that black pills were very good to clean the body.

I was a very mature child, and my aunt and uncle would call me "old lady." They always said I didn't act like a child; I acted like a "big old lady." When I was about twelve years old, I would ride my bicycle to the town's drug store and purchase the black pills for my brother, cousin, and myself. With my aunt's supervision, we would take the black pills. At the time, I felt very good and wise, thinking I was helping my body to be clean. I would dream that one day I would also help many people to be well. So I held onto my dream of being a nurse, healer, and helper to suffering mankind.

During my final year in high school, I knew that my mind was made up to be a nurse. My high school was located in front of the Lucea Hospital in Hanover. I got permission from the boarding house mistress and the matron of the hospital to go to the hospital on Saturdays to obtain insight into the nursing profession (similar experience to the Canadian candy stripers).

I had to board at the school because I lived in another parish, and it was too far to commute to school on a daily basis.

I enjoyed my experience at the hospital, helping to comb the elderly female patients' hair, feeding those who could not feed themselves. I would do anything that was expected of me. I felt like a nurse in training. Two other students who wanted to be nurses accompanied me to the hospital on Saturdays. Today, they also fulfilled their dream of becoming nurses.

After writing my GCE O-levels examination, I applied to the Kingston School of Nursing in Jamaica. I was successful with my examination and was accepted to the school. I left high school in July and commenced nursing training in September of that year.

At the end of the three years' training, I graduated with the director's prize for obtaining the most credits in internal examinations.

Immediately after graduation, I left for Canada to join my mother. Once I arrived in Canada, my mother made arrangements for me to return to high school (O'Neill Collegiate in Oshawa, Ont.) and do grade 13 (having not done A levels in Jamaica, I needed my last year of high school if I had plans to go to university). I obeyed my mother and was enrolled in the grade 13 program. The following year I graduated with my full high school credits.

My mother's friend was the head nurse at the Dr. J. O. Ruddy Hospital in Whitby, Ont., and she got a part-time job for me to work as a graduate nurse pending Canadian registration. I worked on a part-time basis three days per week from 6 pm to 10 pm, gaining Canadian experience. I was still a student at O'Neill Collegiate at that time. I would leave school, go home for a quick bite, and then take the evening bus coming from Bowmanville to Whitby for work three days a week.

After completing high school, I sent my nursing transcript to the College of Nurses of Ontario to obtain my Canadian registration. I received a letter stating I would have to take some continuing education courses for the registered nurses program at Centennial College before writing the examination because I did not have enough hours in some subjects. I was so saddened and I cried for many days. I said to myself: *Imagine, I graduated tops in my nursing class and now they want me to go back to nursing school.* I was now working full time as a graduate nurse pending registration at Dr. J. O. Ruddy Hospital (I think it is now converted into a nursing home).

Although I was not happy with the College of Nursing of Ontario's assessment, I enrolled at Centennial College to upgrade my nurses training to write the nurses registration examination.

After completing my eight-hour tour of duty, working from 7:30 am to 3:30 pm, I would be picked up by another foreign-trained nurse (this lady was trained in England) to attend classes at Centennial College.

Time seemed to have sailed by very fast; I completed the program at Centennial College, wrote my nurses registration examination, and got a job at Toronto Western Hospital. I worked there for one year before accompanying my husband to McMaster University Medical Centre where he was doing his pharmacy residency program. I was fortunate because I also got a job to work in the pharmacy as one of the IV nurses making up intravenous solutions for the neonatal unit and the hospital in general.

After leaving McMaster, we returned to Toronto and I got a job at Humber River Regional Hospital. While working there, I did part-time courses in iridology and natural medicine.

I am very happy to say I have fulfilled my dream by qualifying myself to help suffering humanity.

Nursing Education

- Diploma in nursing from Kingston School of Nursing, 1971.

- Centennial College of Applied Arts and Technology (non-registered graduate nurses program), 1974.
- Seneca College of Applied Arts and Technology, certificate in coronary care nursing, 1981.
- York Finch General Hospital (now Humber River).
- Certificate in nursing assessment skills level 1 and 2, 1981.
- Humber River Regional Hospital, life skills coaches training, 1997.
- Centre for Addiction and Mental Health, psychiatry in the 21st century, certificate of attendance, 2000.

Alternative Medicine Education

- National Iridology Research Association course, 1998.
- Certificate in nutrition and complementary medicine, the Jag Group Irvine, California, 1998.
- Iridology Association of Canada, registered practitioner diploma in clinical iridology, 1999.
- University of Toronto, from evidence to integration, 2001.
- Doctor Nielson's homeopathy education seminar, 2002.
- Clayton College of Natural Health, natural wellness certificate, 2005-2011 (on a part-time basis).
- Alternative Medicine College of Canada, natural health educator diploma, 2010-2011; naturopath diploma, 2011-2012; post-graduate diploma, 2013-2014.
- International Academy of Wellness, certificate in biofeedback, 2013.
- Doctor of Integrative Medicine, Board of Integrative Medicine (World Health Organization), 2014.

Allied Education

- York University, BA in psychology, 1984-1994.

Today, I am a doctor of integrative medicine, specializing in naturopathy and biofeedback. The only regret I have to date is that I did not give back to my country, working as a registered nurse in Jamaica. After I completed my training I was physically tired and wanted a vacation. So I came to Canada to be with my mother. In retrospect, what I should have done was to visit with my mother and return home to study midwifery and give back more to Jamaica before returning to Canada for Canadian registration.

My nursing training in Jamaica was very comprehensive; personally, I think Jamaica trains the best nurses in the world. I think any nurse who was trained in Jamaica can work anywhere, under any condition, anytime. We know how to improvise and we know our work.

CHAPTER TWO

THE BODY

What does a medical professional work with? What is the tool of our profession? The human body? When you think about the body, do the following questions come to mind?

- What is the body?
- What is the body made of?
- How should we treat our bodies?
- How long do we think our bodies will last?
- What will happen if we abuse our bodies?
- What will happen if we take care of our bodies?

What is the body?

The body is like a physical framework with chemical properties that house our organ systems. For this reason, your body in my thinking is likened to a house or a temple. The body is the physical aspect of man.

What is the body made of?

The body is made up of several organ systems, namely:

- digestive;
- respiratory;
- integumentary (skin);
- lymphatic;
- reproductive;
- cardiovascular;
- urinary;
- skeletal;
- nervous;
- muscular.

Each of these systems works in harmony so that the body can function as an integrative unit.

This brief overview of each of the body's systems will help you appreciate your marvelous machine called the body.

THE DIGESTIVE SYSTEM

The digestive system consists of the following:

The mouth is the first part of the digestive system that receives the food we eat. Before the food enters the mouth, the sight and smell of food stimulates the salivary glands to secrete saliva. It hosts the salivary glands, the tongue and the teeth, and is bounded by the lips on the outside.

The salivary glands include three pairs: namely, the parotid, submandibular, and sublingual glands. Saliva is a liquid that pours from these glands to lubricate our food for easier swallowing. Saliva also contains the enzyme amylase that assists in the breakdown of starchy foods.

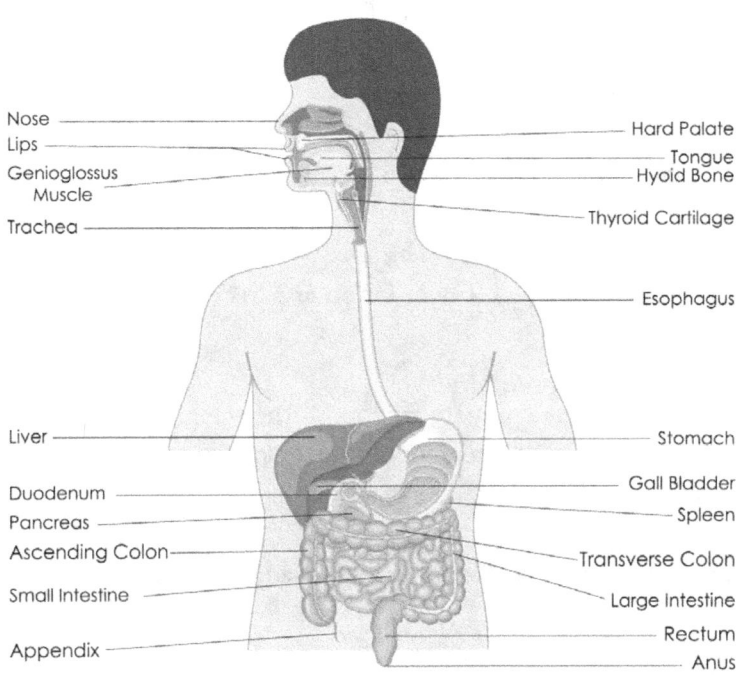

Nose — Hard Palate
Lips — Tongue
Genioglossus — Hyoid Bone
Muscle
Trachea — Thyroid Cartilage

Esophagus

Liver — Stomach
Duodenum — Gall Bladder
Pancreas — Spleen
Ascending Colon — Transverse Colon
Small Intestine — Large Intestine
Rectum
Appendix — Anus

The tongue is made up of several muscles that help to move the food around in the mouth for chewing and swallowing. The tongue has taste buds in different places for four distinct tastes: salty, sour, sweet, and bitter.

The teeth — there are thirty-two in an adult mouth — aid in masticating (chewing and tearing) food, making it easier to swallow. Teeth also help us to speak more clearly.

The esophagus is the tube that carries food from the mouth to the stomach.

The stomach is a muscular cavity that can hold about two quarts of food and drink. Food is temporarily stored in this reservoir for a minimum of three hours before passing on to the small intestines. The stomach is like a chemical station where food-processing takes place thanks to hydrochloric acid and other chemicals that move from the stomach to the small intestines.

Man's **small intestine** is about 6.25 metres long, and is responsible for complete digestion. By the time the chyme leaves the small intestines, all the nourishment has been absorbed or assimilated. In other words, all nutrients have left the GI tract for other parts of the body by the blood stream and the lymph.

The large intestine's primary function is the channel for the elimination of waste matter, and for temporary storage of water, which is reabsorbed into the circulation through the walls of the intestine.

The accessory organs — the **liver, gallbladder** and **pancreas** — are discussed below.

The liver is the largest organ in the body and we could not survive without it. It performs many important bodily functions, including:

- Producing and releasing bile to the gallbladder.
- Breaking down fat molecules with the alkalinity-increasing bile.
- Increasing peristalsis and preventing food from decaying within the digestive tract.
- Giving feces their standard dark yellow-brown colour.
- Storing glycerol and fatty acids to be used as energy.
- Serving as a storehouse and processor for vitamins and minerals — manufacturer of vitamin A.
- Serving as a manufacturing site for cholesterol.

The gallbladder is situated under the right lobe of the liver. It holds about one-and-a-quarter ounces of bile, which is poured into the duodenum when partially digested food enters.

The pancreas is about six inches long and sits at the back of the abdomen behind the stomach. Its function is as follows:

- Pouring the secretions of the insulin and glucagon hormones directly into the bloodstream where they regulate the sugar content.

Every system of the body is very important. But I think the digestive system is the most important. It can be likened to the gas tank of a motor vehicle. The mouth is the body's intake, where the food enters (just as the gas tank takes in gas). Food is broken down, assimilated to help repair worn-out tissue, energize the body, and make the body mobile. If the vehicle doesn't have gas, it will not be able to move; if our bodies don't have the right type of food, there will be a negative impact on the whole system.

THE RESPIRATORY SYSTEM

The respiratory system is composed of:

- the nasal cavity;
- the mouth;
- the larynx;
- the trachea or windpipe;
- the lungs and its structures (bronchi and bronchial tree);
- the rib cage;
- the diaphragm.

Lying behind the breastbone and in front of the heart, the trachea divides into the left and right bronchus, which lead to the left and right lungs.

Air enters the lungs through the nose or the mouth. It passes through the nose and is filtered by hair-like fibres called cilia that are coated with mucus that trap impurities during inhalation. These pollutants return to the trachea for expulsion when we sneeze.

Oxygen is a gas that is vital to the existence of all living cells. It enters our bloodstream from the atmosphere via the respiratory system. Breathing is an automatic action caused by the contraction and relaxation of the diaphragm and other muscles.

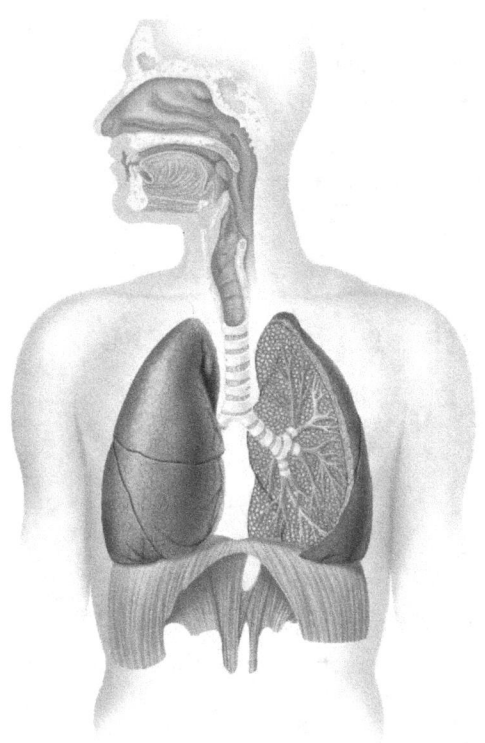

When you inhale, your lungs fill up with air. Oxygen is separated from carbon dioxide and enters the blood and into the capillaries that carry it around the body. At the same time, the blood picks up the carbon dioxide that's produced by the cells and returns it to the lungs where it is exhaled.

THE INTEGUMENTARY SYSTEM (SKIN)

The skin is the largest organ in the body. It covers and protects the body and is made up of two layers: the outer layer, called the epidermis, and the inner layer, called the dermis (the thicker part of the skin). The dermis contains blood vessels, nerves, connective tissues, sweat glands, and sebaceous glands that secrete oil, which lubricates the skin and hair.

When you meet someone for the first time, the first part of your body that impacts them is the skin on your face. This part of the body is thus likened to the front door of the body, which is your house/temple.

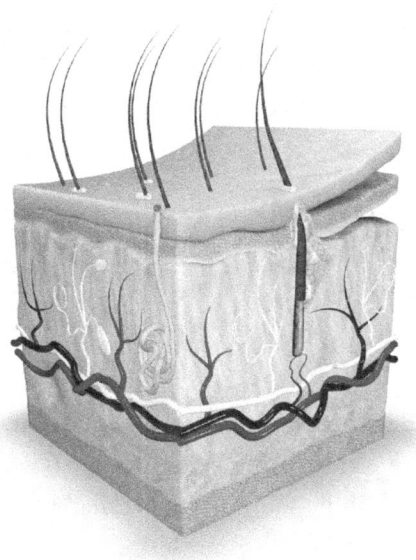

We should take care of our skin and, in particular, our face, like we take care of the exterior of our home. When you see someone's face, you can tell how healthy they are.

Later in the book you will learn more about taking care of the skin.

THE LYMPHATIC SYSTEM

This system is closely related to the circulatory system. It includes lymphatic capillaries, larger vessels, lymph nodes, the spleen, the tonsils, and the thymus. It forms a network of vessels that transports a whitish fluid that is derived from the plasma around the body. Some of this fluid (lymph) seeps through the walls of the capillaries and supplies the areas between individual cells and tissues. Some of the functions of the lymphatic system are as follows:

- Removing disease-causing organisms.
- Manufacturing white blood cells.
- Generating antibodies.
- Distributing fluids and nutrients all over the body (managing the fluid levels in the body), draining off excess fluids and proteins left behind by capillary circulation to prevent swelling of tissues.

THE REPRODUCTIVE SYSTEM

The main purpose of the reproductive system is to create new life. Human beings have male and the female reproductive systems.

The male reproductive system is composed of the scrotum, testes, spermatic ducts, sex glands, and penis. A pair of testes hangs down in the wrinkled bag of skin behind the penis called the scrotum. The testes produce sperm and the male hormone testosterone.

The penis is made of spongy tissues that carry the sperm during copulation. During the sexual act, this spongy tissue is filled with blood, which makes it firmer, forming an erection. The penis also serves as a vessel for urine.

The prostate gland surrounds the urethra and secretes whitish fluid called semen. This fluid carries the spermatozoa during sexual intercourse.

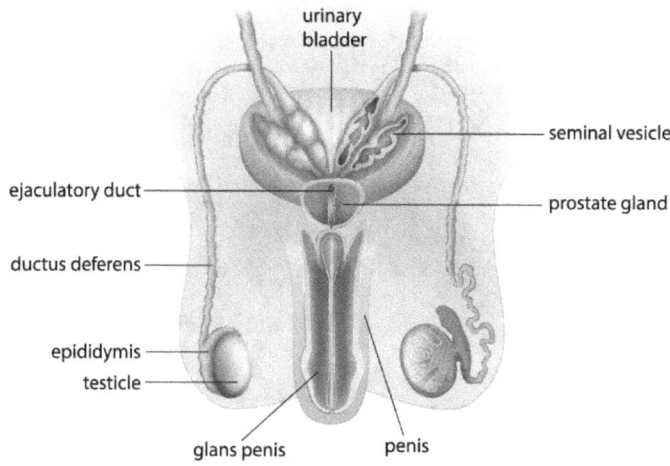

urinary
bladder

seminal vesicle

ejaculatory duct

prostate gland

ductus deferens

epididymis

testicle

glans penis   penis

The female reproductive system consists of the ovaries, fallopian tubes, uterus, vagina, vulva, and mammary glands.

The ovaries are two almond-shaped glands located on each side of the uterus. They secrete hormones that help in female development and produce a large number of eggs (acolytes).

The fallopian tubes (oviducts) are a pair of muscular tubes extending from the corners of the uterus to its edge. When the eggs are released from the ovary, they are swept toward the fallopian tube and transported to the uterus.

The uterus — a hollow muscular pear-shaped organ located posterior and superior to the urinary bladder — is the place where the fertilized ovum is implanted to develop into a baby.

The vagina is a muscular elastic tube that connects the cervix to the uterus to the outside world. It is the canal for the penis during sexual intercourse and it carries the sperm to the uterus.

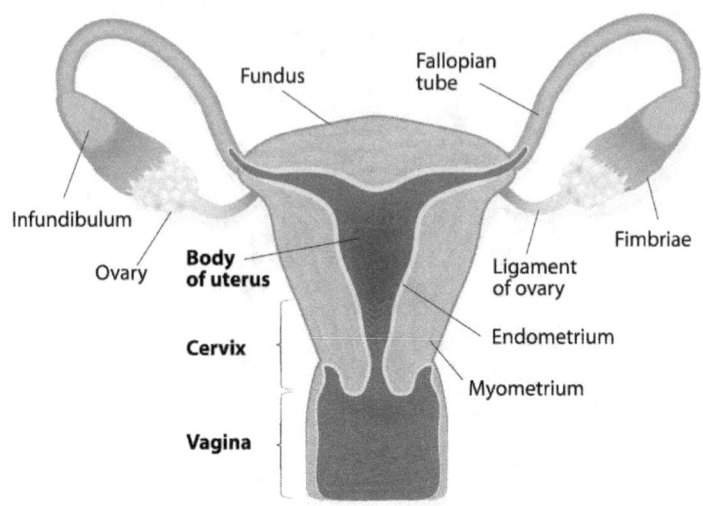

I would like to remind both males and females that your body is the temple of the holy spirit and should not be used for illicit sexual pleasures. You should keep yourselves pure so that you will not have painful regrets in later life. Do not sleep around and think it is cool. Remember: for every action there is a repercussion. Sexual intercourse is a natural part of life. It was meant to facilitate procreation and intimacy between man and wife. If used in the wrong way, it can harm your health and well-being.

What the Bible says about sexual immorality:

- 1 Corinthians 6:18 states: "Flee fornication. Every sin that a man doeth is without the body; but he that committeth fornication sinneth against his own body."
- Hebrews 13:4: "Let marriage be held in honour among all, and let the marriage bed be undefiled, for God will judge the sexually immoral and adulterous."
- Leviticus 18:22: "You shall not lie with a male as with woman; it is an abomination."

- Keep yourself pure and you will live a long, healthy, and happy life.

Some of the consequences of illicit sexual behaviour are as follows:

- Unwanted pregnancies.
- Having abortions with possible complications such as:
  - death due to heavy bleeding or anesthesia failure,
  - uterine perforation,
  - and cancer from hormonal imbalances.
- Dropping out of school.
- Children not getting to know their fathers and feeling confused and angry as a result.
- Getting venereal diseases like herpes, which lasts for a life time.

CARDIOVASCULAR (CIRCULATORY SYSTEM)

The circulatory system is composed of the heart, arteries, veins and capillaries. The heart is a hollow, fist-sized muscular organ located behind the thorax and between the lungs. Its main function is to constantly pump blood around the body, carrying oxygen and glucose and removing waste matter. The blood goes to the lungs first, where it is oxygenated, then to the body via the arteries, where it provides oxygen and carries away waste such as carbon dioxide. From there, it is transported back to the heart for the cycle to begin again.

Blood surrounds and covers all the cells and organs of the body. It is composed of plasma (a pale, watery liquid). Red and white blood cells and platelets float in the plasma. Blood is the carrier of oxygen and nutrients in the form of glucose. It is composed of about 80% water. In the human body, blood is the liquid that surrounds all the tissue, cells, and organs. To me, blood is like a river and all the tissues and organs swim in it. If the river is dirty, then everything in it is dirty. If the river is sluggish, then everything in it moves sluggishly. The average-sized adult has a blood volume of around 4.7 litres. If the blood pressure (the river that is constantly flowing in our blood vessels) is too high, we run the risk of having a stroke or dying; if it is too low, we become dizzy, lightheaded, or can even faint.

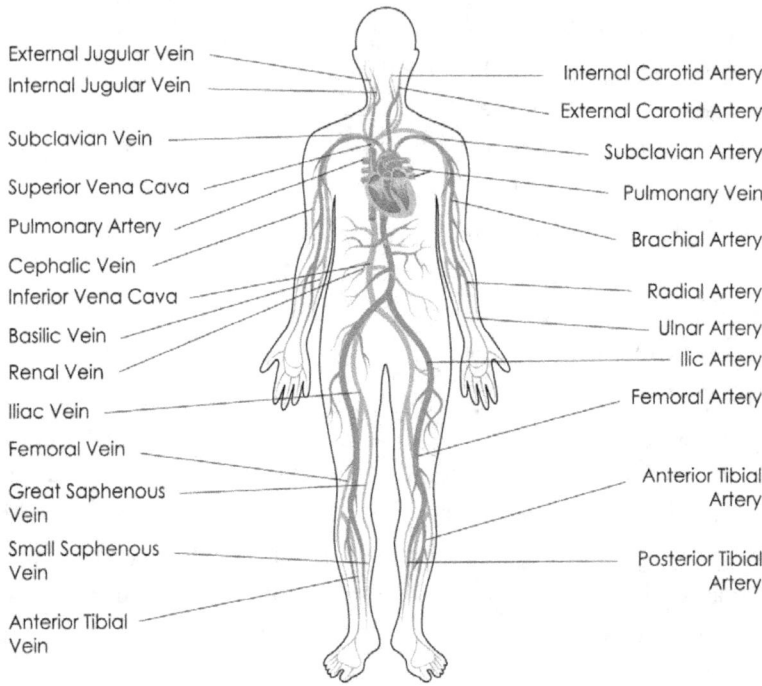

External Jugular Vein
Internal Jugular Vein

Subclavian Vein

Superior Vena Cava

Pulmonary Artery

Cephalic Vein
Inferior Vena Cava

Basilic Vein

Renal Vein

Iliac Vein

Femoral Vein

Great Saphenous Vein

Small Saphenous Vein

Anterior Tibial Vein

Internal Carotid Artery

External Carotid Artery

Subclavian Artery

Pulmonary Vein

Brachial Artery

Radial Artery

Ulnar Artery

Ilic Artery

Femoral Artery

Anterior Tibial Artery

Posterior Tibial Artery

Though some people have no symptoms at all, the more common effects of high blood pressure include the following:

- vision problems;
- shortness of breath;
- headaches;
- dizziness;
- nosebleeds;

- strokes;
- kidney failure.

The effects of low blood pressure include the following:

- dizziness;
- fainting;
- shock;
- kidney failure;
- strokes.

As can be seen from above, low and high blood pressure can have some of the same symptoms. So the most important thing is to try to maintain normal blood pressure.

THE URINARY SYSTEM

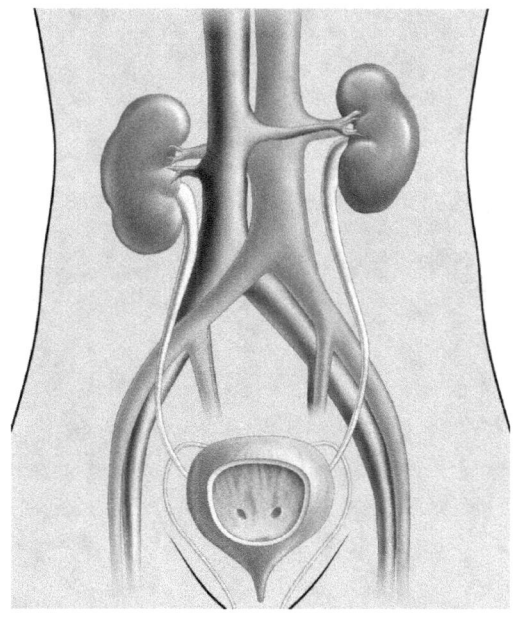

The urinary system is made of the kidneys, ureters, urinary bladder, and urethra. The kidneys are a pair of bean-shaped organs located behind the abdominal cavity on either side of the spine. They exist to:

- help purify our body by filtering the blood to remove waste.
- regulate the amount of fluid in the body.
- regulate the salt content in the blood.
- regulate the acid-alkaline balance of the blood.

THE MUSCULAR AND SKELETAL SYSTEM

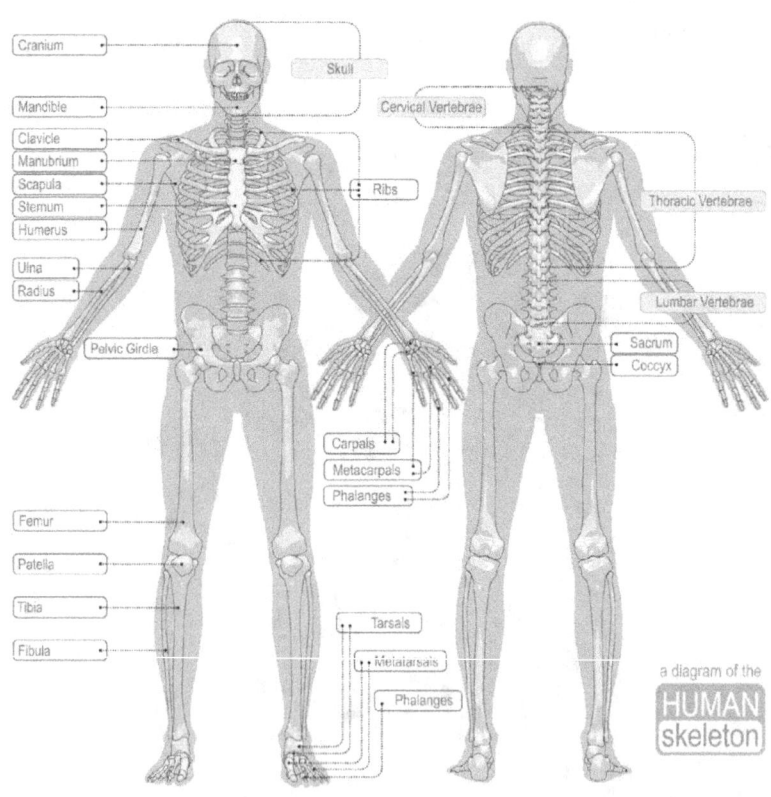

The skeletal system forms the framework of the body and protects all our internal organs. For example, the skull bones protect the delicate brain; the ribs protect the heart and lungs. This bony framework also allows us to stand and walk. The bones and muscles work as a team to facilitate most of our movements. Adults have 206 bones. Babies have 305 bones but, as they grow, they become fused together to make larger bones.

Our bones become more brittle as the human skeleton ages. If the diet is lacking in calcium and other minerals, the bones can weaken over time. Wear and tear of the bones and joints can also cause problems in the long run.

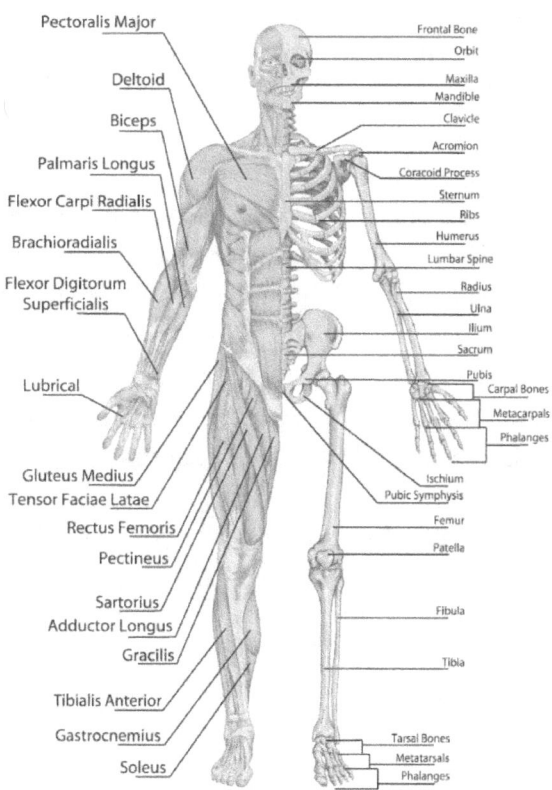

THE NERVOUS SYSTEM AND BRAIN

The nervous system — composed of the brain, spinal cord, and cranial nerves — is a marvellous network system controlled by the brain. The delicate mass of tissues called the brain is protected by the skull and meninges (strong fibrous membranes). It has three main parts:

- The cerebrum is the largest and most developed part of the human brain. Divided into right and left hemispheres, it is responsible for the conscious and voluntary aspect of our existence (thinking, learning, memory). It receives and translates sensory stimuli and helps to control our motor functions.
- The cerebellum is the section of the brain that is behind and below the cerebrum. It has two lateral lobes and a middle lobe. Its main function is concerned with managing the muscular functions of the body and the unconscious functions. It also helps to maintain equilibrium (balance).
- The brain stem is composed of three parts: the mid brain, the pons, and the medulla oblongata, the section of the brain responsible for those bodily functions that happen automatically, such as eye movements, respiration, heart rate, swallowing, coughing, body temperature, and sexual arousal. These are all functions of the automatic nervous system as opposed to the central nervous system.
- The spinal cord is a thick cord of nerve tissue of the central nervous system. It is also the main path that connects information between the brain and peripheral nervous system.
- Cranial nerves are comprised of twelve pairs that derive from the brain and brain stem and are responsible for sensory and motor functions, including:

    1. Olfactory nerve — sensory/smell
    2. Optic nerve — sensory/sight
    3. Oculomotor — motor/muscles of the eye
    4. Trochlear — motor/muscles of the eye

5. Trigeminal — mixed/teeth, skin, face, head
6. Abducent — motor/eye
7. Facial — mixed/expression of face; sensory/tongue
8. Auditory — sensory/hearing
9. Glosso-pharyngeal — mixed/taste, muscles of pharynx)
10. Vagus — mixed/larynx, pharynx, heart, spleen, lungs, esophagus, liver, stomach, pancreas
11. Spinal accessory — mixed/neck muscles and viscera
12. Hypoglossal — mixed/tongue muscles

The brain is considered the governing centre of the body, and if it's not functioning properly, it can manifest in many different types of behaviour. I will discuss some common conditions that can affect the brain later in the book.

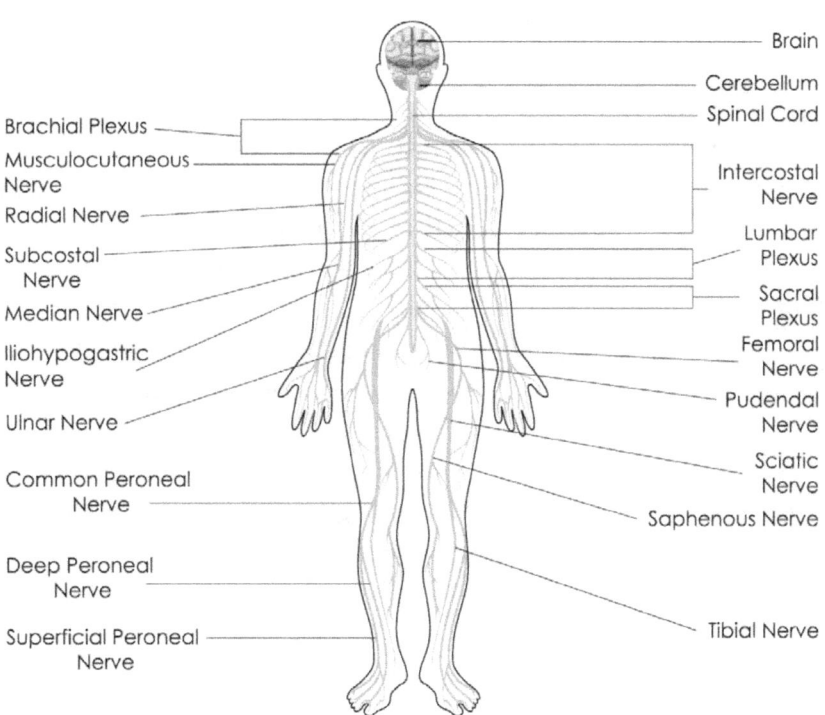

CHAPTER THREE

LIFE, THE PERFECT GIFT

After describing the perfectly made specimen called the body, whose component parts I briefly outlined above, I am agreeing with Genesis 2:7 that states, "Then the Lord God formed the man of dust from the ground and breathed into his nostrils the breath of life, and the man became a living creature." It's clear to me that the human body is indeed a temple, made by the hands of God. As such, shouldn't we keep it clean? Why then do we dump garbage inside this marvellous specimen? Let us make a conscious effort to treat this perfect gift with the respect it's due. The time is now. We are not promised tomorrow so, as they commonly say in Jamaica, let's "make hay while the sun still shines." In other words, let's do what we have to do while we can still see and while it is daylight. Let us take care of our bodies. Let us take responsibility for our own health. If we do, it will pay off as we grow older.

Many health problems rarely have a single cause or a single solution. Most conditions arise from a multitude of factors, including:

- diet;
- stress levels;
- exercise habits;

- supplements you take (or don't take);
- relationship problems.

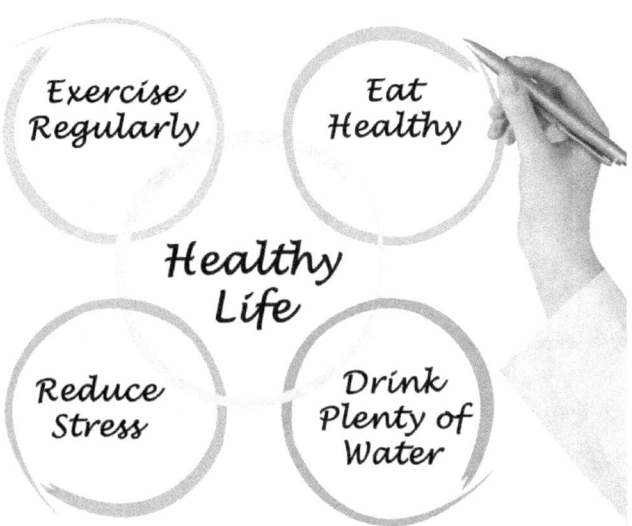

In this book, we will offer a multitude of suggestions to help you take responsibility for your health.

Life is a perfect gift that we should not take for granted. Good health is a special bonus to our life. As a registered nurse looking back on my career, I have seen so much suffering and pain that could have been avoided had the sufferers only taken the time to realize how precious their life and health were, had they only taken responsibility for what they put in their bodies and how they live their lives.

Remember, life on this earth is very brief, so we have to spend our time wisely. And the wisest approach is to take responsibility for your health, in order to have a good life. You should always bear in your mind that your life is not a game. It's not a play rehearsal. It is your sole opportunity to go through this cycle on earth. Life is meant to be taken seriously, so try your best to do things right and take responsibility for your health.

This book will give you a little understanding of your current health so that you can improve not just the length, but the quality, of your life and that of your family. When you have good health and vitality, you will have the energy to pursue anything. Taking care of your health is very important all the time, but even more important as you grow older. It's critical to have a family doctor who can give you guidance when you're not feeling well and refer you to specialists and other investigative channels as required.

Look around and you will see people everywhere who are looking for solutions and answers to ease their diseases and disabilities. Increasingly, they begin to realize that much of the morbidity and mortality in Western society relates to their *lifestyle*, especially our rich Western diet. We are bombarded with many different reports and studies about today's diet, which consists of fast foods, processed foods, and a lack of fruits and vegetables. My past diet is a typical example. When you are busy, it is very difficult to spend the time to prepare healthy meals, and we are oftentimes tempted to purchase fast foods, which are processed.

If we desire to keep our bodies — life's perfect gift — healthy, we will have to give up eating junk food. These are foods that are high in sugar, salt, fat, and calories, and have little nutritional value. Some of these foods include the following:

- gum;
- snack foods such as chips, cookies, and candies;
- desserts;
- fried foods (French fries);
- carbonated beverages;
- hamburgers, pizza, and tacos.

Ingesting this addictive, enticing food is like throwing garbage (leftover food) down the kitchen pipes. It provides too much fat and calories, and has been linked to serious health problems. If you throw garbage down your kitchen pipes, the pipes will become blocked; if you put junk food (too much fat and calories) in your body, your veins and arteries will become blocked. Let's take a closer look and see some of the harm eating junk food can do to our bodies:

- By consuming more fat and calories, you are at risk of being obese.
- Consuming junk food over a period of time will cause a continuous rapid rise in blood sugar. This will cause a chronically high insulin level, ultimately leading to obesity and type 2 diabetes.
- Because junk food consists of large amounts of simple carbo-hydrates, a sudden drop in blood sugar is also evident (because of inadequate protein) after eating. This gives rise to low energy, fatigue, and a craving for more sugar.
- Depression is a change in hormone levels from consuming trans fat, especially in young adults.
- High blood pressure, which can lead to heart disease.
- Altered brain activity similar to that which results from cocaine and heroin use (research done at Scripps Research Institute).

Now that you have a glimpse into the world of junk food, I think you should make a conscious effort to seriously evaluate what you put into your mouth. Remember, you only have one life, and what you do with it will determine how you will spend your golden years.

Allopathic (pharmaceutical) doctors do not have the time to care for the whole person; their major concerns are to relieve the immediate symp-toms. To obtain a cure and proper therapy, we have to go the seat of the problem. We have to find the cause of the problem before we can correct it. Let's examine the total makeup of mankind. There are three distinct aspects to every human being, namely:

- physical;
- psychological;
- spiritual.

Most times, we wait until the body gives us warning signals before even visiting a doctor. By then, it is often too late. I have a sign posted in my office that says, "Take responsibility for your health before it is too late." We all want to be well, to be healthy. Let us examine the concept of wellness.

WELLNESS

Wellness encompasses physical, psychological, and social stability. In this state, there is no disease and the individual can cope mentally and adjust to social settings. It involves the following:

- the whole person with a positive approach to life;
- physical health;
- emotional health;
- spiritual health;
- social health.

CHAPTER FOUR

HOMEOSTASIS AND THE BODY

My approach to this topic, *Taking Responsibility for Your Own Health,* is to highlight the effects of:

- homeostasis and the body.
- the condition of body chemistry (chemical imbalance and how it affects the body's systems).
- high acidity in the system and its effect on all the bodily systems.
- stress.
- your risk factors.

HOMEOSTASIS

Homeostasis is maintaining internal balance within the body's organs. This involves the following:

- Regulating the body's temperature.
- Having a balanced pH system (stability between acidity/alkalinity).
- A constant environment for the internal body chemistry.

According to Nancy Appleton, PhD, "in human beings, homeostasis commonly referred to the internal balance of the body's electromagnetic and chemical systems." When this balance is maintained, we have the right amount of hormones in the blood and other organs.

An overstressed body, however, will not function correctly and will not be in a state of homeostasis. One of the biggest barriers to homeostasis is our modern-day lifestyle.

Living in the 21st century is a major problem with the human race. We are blessed with an advanced way of life, and our work is so much easier than that of our forefathers who were hunters and gatherers. In our advanced technological world, most of our supplies are ready-made — and it's killing us. We overeat, and we consume more sugar and fat than we did in the past. These overindulgences are causing physical turmoil and wrecking our immune systems. We do everything in excess.

There are so many fast-food restaurants in our society compared to developing societies. At almost every intersection in our major cities there are fast-foods outlets. The McDonald's food chains are all over the globe. They are selling millions of French fries, hamburgers, and milkshakes on a daily basis. Consuming this type of diet (high fat and calories) on a regular basis will only block the arteries. We are on a slow slope to killing ourselves.

Our supermarkets are filled with processed foods: canned goods, frozen goods, and foods in packages. In order to keep these products viable, many chemicals are added to them. Unfortunately, our system is not equipped to digest them.

Our allopathic doctors are prescribing more and more prescriptions for their clients. What can these poor doctors do? If the clients visit them and are not given a prescription or two, they are upset; sometimes even saying that the doctor is not good for not prescribing any drugs. Yes, people go to their doctor looking for a quick fix with a magic pill. What they do not understand is that these so-called magic pills are Band-Aid therapy, hiding the real cause of their problems. In the long run, they are poison to the system. Yes, we are programmed to believe we need a magic pill to fix every ailment.

HOW TO FIND OUT IF YOUR BODY IS NOT IN HOMEOSTASIS

First, start by listening to your body. Our bodies give us warning signals long before something serious happens to us. You may have symptoms that won't go away, (this is when the body is giving us warning signals), and sometimes your doctor, or magic pill, is not able to help you. Here are some signs and symptoms that all is not well with us. If you do not heed the warning signals that the body gives us, the body will start to scream (this is when we will have a full-blown disease). Symptoms will be divided into different categories and can be exhibited if your system is alkaline or acidic. Some of the symptoms are as follows:

GASTROINTESTINAL

Anorexia, binge eating, bloating, canker sores, indigestion, nausea, nervous stomach, irritable colon, diarrhea, gas, constipation, hunger between meals, vomiting.

CENTRAL NERVOUS SYSTEM

Nervousness, fatigue, anxiety, depression, hyperactivity, confusion, dizziness, drowsiness, headache, hostility, irritability, mood change, insomnia, high blood pressure, low blood pressure, fullness of the head.

MUSCULOSKELETAL

Muscle aches, muscles cramps, swelling, stiffness, back pain, joint pain, knee pain.

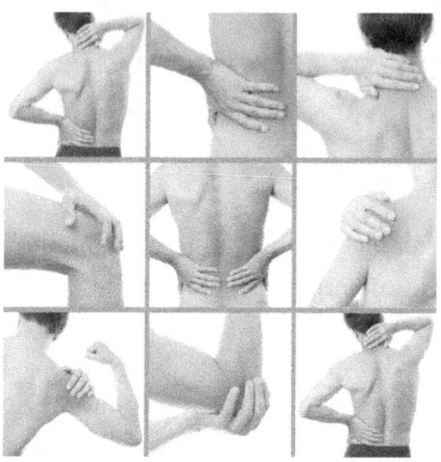

RESPIRATORY

Asthma, hay fever, sinusitis, runny nose, scratchy throat, itchy ears, coughing, sneezing.

CIRCULATORY

Irregular heartbeat, increased heartbeat, palpitations, dark circles under the eyes, high blood pressure, low blood pressure, swollen ankles and wrists.

SKIN

Hives, rashes, acne, psoriasis, edema, eczema, unusual skin pallor, dryness, wrinkles.

GYNECOLOGICAL

Vaginal discharge, vaginal itching, PMS, menopausal symptoms, menstrual cramps, swollen breasts, breast lumps.

OTHER

Candida albicans, Epstein-Barr virus, chronic fatigue, fibromyalgia, falling asleep after meals, water retention, hyperglycemia, hypoglycemia, environmental illness.

Some of the most common symptoms that warn you that something is not right are: headaches, fatigue, joint pain, lower back pain, and falling asleep after meals.

SYSTEMIC ACIDOSIS

Many studies have shown that most people who have unbalanced pH are "acidic." Most of the clients I see are acidic, so let's focus on high acidity in the body.

High acidity in the body is another form of chemical imbalance and can affect all major body systems, such as:

the digestive system
 • Gastric ulcers, stomach aches, nausea, vomiting, burning discomfort in the stomach.

the intestinal system
 • Constipation or diarrhea.

the circulatory system
 • Chest pain, swollen ankles.

the respiratory system
- chronic airway problems;
- asthma;
- shortness of breath.

the immune system
- weakness, susceptible to infections.

the nervous system
- depression of the central nervous system
- anxiety and nervousness

the glandular system
- diabetic acidosis (breath smells fruity), confusion.

the urinary system
- bladder and kidney problems.

the structural system
- fatigue and muscle stiffness, lack of calcium can cause muscle spasms and twitching, tension in the neck and shoulders, arthritis, and osteoporosis

the growth of cancer cells
- cancer cells are abnormal growths that can survive in an acidic, anoxic condition.

Our bodies were created to be alkaline by our creator, but many of its functions are acidic. When Albert Szent-Györgyi discovered vitamin C, he realized that. For this reason, in order to maintain proper health, the body must neutralize or excrete a large amount of the acid it produces. Acid-alkaline balance is one of the essential criteria for optimum health.

According to the Dorland's Medical Dictionary, pH 7 is neutral. In other words, it is neither acidic nor alkaline. Above seven is more alkaline; below seven its acidity increases.

In order to help people overcome an acid imbalance, we will have to take a more indepth view on the acid-alkaline issue by examining the following:

- How does an acid-alkaline imbalance promote diseases?
- How do you determine whether food will produce more acid in the body?
- How can supplementing our diet accelerate vibrant health?
- How do you measure acid and alkaline in our body?
- How do you keep the balance right for optimum health?

HOW TO MEASURE ACID AND ALKALINE IN OUR BODIES

Measuring the acid-alkaline balance of your system can be easily done in the comfort of your home.If your pH level stays between 6.4 and 6.8 all day, your body is functioning normally. The best time to test your pH is about one hour before, and two hours after, a meal. Check your pH twice weekly by using NSP (Nature's Sunshine Products) pH strips. You will be able to determine the status of your pH. If your urine pH fluctuates between 6.0 and 6.4 in the morning, and 6.4 and 7.0 in the evening, your body is functioning normally.

HOW CAN SUPPLEMENTING OUR FOOD ACCELERATE CHANGES IN OUR BODIES?

Taking supplements and medication can cause the system to be either acid or alkaline. It has been proven that most synthetic vitamins are acidifying. One of the most acidifying of all is ascorbic acid.

ACID PRODUCTION IS NATURAL

Let's take a look at the function of hydrochloric acid in the stomach. "Hydrochloric acid is a corrosive substance, and except in very diluted strength, can eat away the lining of the stomach." Hydrochloric acid in the stomach is diluted by mucus secretion that makes it normal and harmless. The normality of the stomach is still acidic, which serves to inhibit the growth of organisms such as bacteria (*Medical and Health Encyclopedia*).

CHAPTER FIVE

THE CHIP PROGRAM

In 2007, I attended the four-week Complete Health Improvement Program (CHIP) program in Toronto, and was impacted in the most powerful and positive way. The program certainly changed my life in many healthy ways. While writing this book, I contacted Dr. Hans A. Diehl to get permission to share some of the information I learned at that program. His reply was, "Spread it around. Best wishes. Go for it." As you read some of the health nuggets, I suggest that you try to register for the CHIP program when it returns to Toronto.

In his lectures and books, Dr. Diehl emphasizes that "people can do more for their health than any doctor, hospital, or technological advancement." This statement is so powerful because if people would simply listen to what their bodies are telling them and respond appropriately, they could save themselves so many heartaches and pain. The choices you make in life will impact your health.

New research is showing the benefit of integrative medicine. Nutrition is playing an ever-increasing role in complementary medicine. Dr. Diehl has a CHIP program that claims we can "reverse disease with a fork and knife." That simply means that if you eat the right type of foods, it can heal your body. In Genesis 1:29, God said, "See, I have given you every herb that yields seed which is on the face of all the earth, and every tree whose fruit yields seed; to you it shall be for food." As many doctors struggle with quality of life and how to help their patients — especially those with chronic degenerative diseases — they look to nutritional support to help offset the effects of medications. They are now learning and appreciating that the body needs necessary nutrients to support the immune system, the endocrine system, and the process of energy metabolism.

Dr. Diel states, "To win the battle against the epidemic of Western lifestyle diseases, we must break with the lethal excesses of today's American diet. We need a simpler, more natural way to eat." Hippocrates, the father of medicine, states, "Let nutrition be your medicine."

One would think that with the advent of industrialization and the advancement of science and new technology, our Western civilization would not be plagued with so many chronic degenerative diseases. That is not the case. In our capitalistic society, the big multinational corporations are all trying to make big bucks, and one of the fastest ways to do this is by selling food. Human beings cannot live without food. But our lifestyles and the type of food we eat are killing us.

Albert Einstein once said, "Nothing happens until something moves." He was speaking of science, but he might as well have been referring to our lifestyle and eating habits. Most people are imprisoned by a lack of effort to improve their state. The only way to break free is to take responsibility for your health. Here's how to revitalize your life and take action the smart way.

The central philosophy of a healthy and happy life

- Know the reason you are doing what you are doing.
- Create a wellness plan.
- The state of wellness is being in good health, not just the absence of disease.

- A positive approach to living, which involves:
  - the whole person;
  - physical;
  - psychological;
  - spiritual well-being;
- responding to your body's warning signals before something serious happens;
- resting well;
- exercise.

KNOW THE REASON YOU ARE DOING WHAT YOU ARE DOING

Maybe you would like to lose some weight. Maybe you want more energy so you can feel healthier, fitter, and younger. Maybe you are worried about developing a degenerative disease that afflicts your family, or perhaps you are suffering from a chronic illness and want to be less dependent on allopathic drugs. Regardless of your reason or concern, this information should be of some assistance to you. You may have heard of Tony Robbins and his work, which states that "no matter what goal you set, the more reasons you have for achieving it, the more you'll convince yourself of wanting to complete it, and you'll go out and get it." So answer these questions and commence your journey.

- Why do you want to get healthy now and not before now?
- What has caused this motivation?
- How committed are you?

Don't be afraid to take responsibility for your life. You can do it. People can do anything if they are committed. Make some lifestyle changes and prepare to see the difference in your life. When you have a clear idea of how much food to eat, when to eat and where to eat, the next and most important step is to look at what you are going to eat. It is never too late to change your eating habits and start taking responsibility for your health. Now that you know what to do, let's get started with your goal of living a healthier, happier, and more fulfilled life.

CREATE A WELLNESS PLAN

Wellness does not only include physical health (nutrition, exercise, weight management, etc.), but every aspect of your life. You should take a holistic view of yourself and how you intend to live the rest of your life. To live your life to the fullest is not a one-day fix, and it's not something you start doing once you visit a doctor. It is something you do on a daily basis. Take the time to get to know more about you, your health issues, your medications, your medical tests, and food that may make you sick; in short, **become an expert on you.**

"The unexamined life is not worth living," Socrates said at his trial for heresy. He was on trial for encouraging his students to challenge the accepted beliefs of the time and think for themselves. Set aside time to:

- examine your life.
- choose your destination.
- choose what you want for yourself, your future.

When you have a clear idea of who you are and what you want from life, you can set your goals. There should be a time in everyone's life to examine their life and strive for a healthier one. You should review your past and make conscious efforts to improve yourself. Take a holistic approach to wellness and concentrate on what you put in your mouth, and in your mind and your spirit. The goal is to aim for a balance in all areas of your life, to help transform the quality of your life so that you can live happier, longer, and healthier.

Your greatest accomplishment in this life should be striving to be "the very best you were created to be," starting with taking responsibility for your health. Find a vision for your life, and work on this vision or dream. In order to focus correctly on this vision, you will need good health.

When setting up a wellness plan or **taking control of your health**, your focus should be on a preventative regime. Thomas Edison once said, "The doctor of the future will give no medicine but will interest his patients in the care of the human frame, *in diet and the cause and prevention of disease.*"

Your wellness plan should incorporate some of the following:

PHYSICAL STATE

- Your energy level – Are you feeling energetic or tired and run down?
- Are you getting a good night's sleep or are you having restless, sleepless nights?
- Are you satisfied with your weight?
- Are you getting enough exercise?
- Is your diet balanced?

SOCIAL HEALTH

- Do you have a social outlet? Do you have time to spend with friends or relatives, like going to the movies or out to eat?

SPIRITUAL HEALTH

- This is a personal journey between you and the creator. It is your responsibility to go to church, the temple, or the synagogue if you so desire.
- You can pray or meditate in your own quiet time whenever you desire.

- However, it is a good thing to examine the spiritual aspect of your life to find out where you fit in and where you are going.

EMOTIONAL HEALTH

I spent the last ten years of my nursing career working as a psychiatric nurse and some of the most important things I would emphasize to my clients were:

- Stress is a natural part of life. It can be good stress or bad stress. It can keep us motivated, or it can destroy us.
- Regular exercise or deep breathing exercise can help our emotional state by helping us to relax.
- Listening to relaxing music also helps our emotional state.
- Getting the right amount of sleep (seven to nine hours per night) is important.
- Keep a journal. This will help you express what is going on inside. Writing about stressful events can help to relieve intra-psychic tension and put many things in proper perspective.

ENVIRONMENTAL HEALTH

According to the World Health Organization, environmental health addresses all the physical, chemical, and biological factors around us. In addition, it is aimed at preventing illness.

It is your responsibility to control some of the environmental factors around you, to make your life healthier.

If you live in a tropical country prone to infections from mosquito bites, make sure there are no breeding grounds for mosquitoes around.

INTELLECTUAL WELLNESS

Living in North America, everyone should try to stimulate their brains. There is so much opportunity in this country for intellectual growth that no one should be left behind. Everyone should be able to read; if not, he or she should seek out some form of mental stimulation.

OCCUPATIONAL WELLNESS

If you can work, you should go to work. You should be in a job that gives you some satisfaction and pride. For this reason, you should choose a job that you enjoy because you will be there for most of the week, and if you are not happy that will impact on your health.

PREVENTIVE HEALTH

Preventive health care is about dealing with conditions before they manifest themselves in a disease or disorder. It is about maintaining health rather than dealing with disease. The World Health Organization has stated that at least 85% of all diseases are preventable. Today in the UK and North America, one in every two deaths is caused by heart disease and circulatory diseases, and one in every four is caused by cancer. Diabetes continues to increase at a rapid rate, with children more likely to become diabetic than their parents.

In fact, all chronic degenerative diseases are increasing at alarming rates, mainly because we refuse to acknowledge a simple law of health and disease: the law of cause and effect. We reap only that which we have sown. If you keep living the wrong way, eating the wrong type of food, not getting enough sleep you may well succumb to disease. According to Galatians 6:7, "Be not deceived: God is not mocked: for whatever a man soweth, that shall he also reap." I think that simply means that everything you do will have an effect on your life. You will reap the consequences of all your actions. If you eat too much junk food, it will affect you negatively one day.

THE LAW OF CAUSE AND EFFECT

The law of cause and effect states that everything happens for a reason. All actions have consequences and produce specific results, as do all inactions. This simply means that you will reap whatever you sow.

Our bodies can self-heal. This life force was given to us from birth to keep us healthy and to heal us in times of distress. Part of our healing force consists of the white blood cells (leucocytes) that travel through the bloodstream, destroying invading bacteria. However, many people compromise this healing energy by eating refined foods with lots of white sugar. In the long term, these will have catastrophic consequences on our healing force and state of health. For this reason, in order to be healthy, we must avoid things that destroy the healing energy and do those things that strengthen and encourage a strong and active healing within our bodies.

WELLNESS

We have to keep in mind that "wellness is the pursuit of continued growth and balance in the seven (aspects) of wellness," namely:

PHYSICAL WELLNESS

- Body

EMOTIONAL WELLNESS (MENTAL)

- Feelings

ENVIRONMENTAL WELLNESS

- Air
- Water
- Safety

SOCIAL WELLNESS

- Family
- Friends
- Relationships

OCCUPATIONAL WELLNESS

- Career
- Skills

INTELLECTUAL WELLNESS

- Mind

SPIRITUAL WELLNESS

- Value
- Purpose
- Intuition
- Vitality

PHYSICAL WELLNESS

To sum up physical wellness, we would have to address all the following:

- Abstaining from harmful habits such as smoking, drinking alcohol, and taking illicit drugs.

- Getting regular medical check-ups.
- Protecting yourself from injuries and harm.
- Daily exercise.
- Getting adequate rest.
- Learning to recognize early signs of illness.
- Practicing safe sex.
- Eating a variety of healthy foods.

In the fifth century B.C., Hippocrates, the godfather of Western medicine, advised people to "let food be your medicine and medicine be your food." This idea is not much in fashion in the West today, but it is strikingly current in Asia. In both India and China, highly developed systems of healing and cuisine are intertwined. Consider:

- We have to eat to live.
- Eating is a major source of pleasure.
- Food that is healthy and food that gives pleasure are not mutually exclusive.
- Eating is an important focus of social interaction.
- How we eat reflects and defines our personal and cultural identity.
- How we eat is a determinant of health.
- Changing how we eat is one strategy for managing disease and restoring health.

There is not a particular diet for the treatment of heart disease, another diet for obesity, another for diabetes, and another for hypertension or osteoporosis. Instead, there is **ONE OPTIMAL DIET.**

This type of diet should comprise different foods and should be eaten when you need it. It should be prepared simply, not using trans fats, heavy oils, sugars, or salt. This food should have no preservatives.

This simpler, more natural dietary lifestyle brings improved health and increased energy. It also allows you to eat larger portions of food while cutting down on your grocery bills. With increasing numbers of heart attacks every year and the rising numbers of cancers internationally, I think it's time we seriously start to think of changing our diets.

During the CHIP program, the following information was emphasized:

EAT LESS:

- **Fats and oils** (avoid fatty meats).
- **Sugars** (limit sugar, honey, molasses).
- **Foods containing cholesterol** (strictly limit meat, sausages, egg yolks, and liver; also, limit dairy products).
- **Salt** (don't salt food during cooking or at the table).
- **Alcohol** (avoid alcohol in all forms, as well as caffeinated beverages such as coffee, colas, and black tea).

EAT MORE:

- **Whole grains** (freely use brown rice, millet, barley, corn, wheat, and rye).
- **Tubers and legumes** (freely use all kinds of white potatoes, sweet potatoes, and yams).
- **Fruits and vegetables** (eat several fresh whole fruits every day).
- **Water** (drink six to eight glasses of water a day; vary the routine with a twist of lemon and occasional herb teas).
- **Hearty breakfasts** (enjoy hot multigrain cereals, fresh fruit, and whole-wheat toast).

MOST DANGEROUS CULPRITS:

1. Salt
2. Sugar
3. Fat

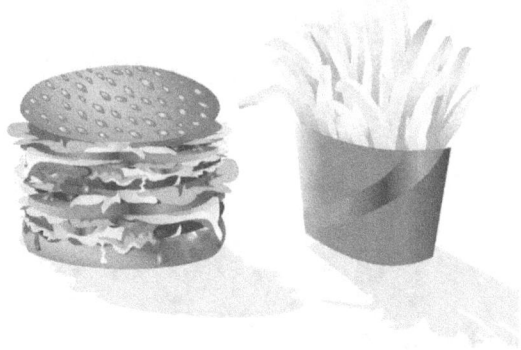

Make the appropriate changes to avoid the hidden ingredients to reduce your risk of diseases.

SPECIAL NOTE ON SALT

Salt, also known as sodium chloride (NaCl), is essential for life. It adds flavour to our food and has two very important functions in our bodies:

1. Regulates the fluid balance.
2. Controls the electrical signals of the nervous system.

Excessive salt be very bad, because it causes the system to retain fluid. This can be seen in swollen ankles and wrists. It puts extra pressure on the heart and can lead to strokes.

SPECIAL NOTE ON SUGAR

Sugar is a sweet carbohydrate substance found naturally in most plants and used as food. Many of us have a sweet tooth that always craves sugar.

Many of us do not know the danger this sweet "devil" poses to our bodies. Let's examine some of the negative and positive effects of sugar. It:

- promotes tooth decay;
- makes you hyperactive, especially young children;
- makes some people more anxious and depressed;
- raises fasting blood sugar and may contribute to diabetes;
- contributes to weight gain/obesity;
- causes headaches/migraines in some people;
- contributes to some forms of cancer;
- makes food tastier;
- boosts energy.

SPECIAL NOTE ON WATER

Approximately 70% of our body's mass is made of water and, according to a number of doctors, drinking eight glasses daily fulfills the necessary requirement of this liquid demand from our bodies. No living thing can live without this tasteless, odourless liquid. For the human body, it is used both internally as well as externally. Here are some of the many benefits of water. It:

- cleans the skin in bathing.
- makes the hair clean and healthy.
- quenches the thirst.
- hydrates the inside of the body, making the skin smooth and firm.
- flushes toxins from the body and helps to relieve constipation.
- helps to prevent headaches (because your brain is about 90% water), and relieves dehydration.
- helps to promote weight loss.
- keeps the joints lubricated, thereby cutting down on joint pain.

SPECIAL NOTE ON FAT

Fat is a necessary part of our diet, like proteins and carbohydrates. But there are good fats and bad fats. Good fats come from fish and vegetable products, and they are called polyunsaturated and monounsaturated fats. Polyunsaturated fats can be found in nuts, seeds, fish, and leafy green vegetables. Monounsaturated fats include mostly plant-based liquid oils such as canola oils, olive oils, peanut oils, safflower oils, and sesame oils, as well as avocados, many nuts, and seeds. Some of the benefits of mono-unsaturated and polyunsaturated fats are:

- They lower bad cholesterol.
- They reduce the risk of heart attack and stroke.
- They promote weight loss.

A SPECIAL NOTE ON CARBOHYDRATES

Carbohydrates are another important food group. They are also called starches and sugars and can be found in grains, fruits, and vegetables. There are two types of carbohydrates:

1. Simple carbohydrates. These are carbohydrates that give you quick energy. They are naturally occurring sugars in a variety of fruits, some vegetables, honey, and maple sap. Processed sugars include table sugar, brown sugar, and molasses.
2. Complex carbohydrates. Your body needs these important starches and fibres. You get them from grains, bread, pastas, and vegetables such as white and sweet potatoes, corn, and dried beans. Our digestive system lacks the enzymes and organisms needed to break down most fibres, including cellulose and other woody parts of the plants. But dietary fibre is still necessary and important because it promotes smooth colon function and may help to prevent colon cancer.

SUPPLEMENTING YOUR DIET

In our fast-paced society, many people do not have the time to eat a proper, home-cooked meal, and they are always on the go. These people are not eating a wide variety of foods and their bodies may be lacking in vital nutrients. In this case, it is advisable for them to supplement their diet with vitamins and minerals.

VITAMINS AND MINERALS

Vitamins are organic substances (made by plants or animals). Minerals are inorganic elements that come from the earth. Animals and humans absorb minerals from the plants they eat. Vitamins and minerals are nutrients that our bodies need to grow and develop normally. Vitamins and minerals have a unique role to play in maintaining your health. Vitamins have antioxidant qualities and help protect the immune system from free radicals. Let's examine some of the vitamins and see what benefits they will add to our diet.

Vitamin A protects against infections. Deficiency of this vitamin leads to night blindness. Some of the foods rich in vitamin A are carrots, sweet potatoes, dark leafy greens, squash, pumpkins, and romaine lettuce.

Vitamin E has many functions. The most important is its antioxidant function, in which it acts as a scavenger, preventing the formation of free radicals in the tissues. It also has some blood-thinning properties that help to dissolve blood clots and keep the arteries clean. Some foods rich in vitamin E are nuts, seeds, avocados, vegetable oils, and wheat germ.

Vitamin C plays a role with the connective tissues of the body. This is a water-soluble vitamin that helps with the following:

- preventing colds;
- increasing the speed of wound healing;
- lowering cholesterol.

B vitamins protect both the immune and nervous systems. They help build blood, protect the body against infection, and produce antibodies. They increase the production of hydrochloric acid for digestion and are vital in helping stabilize mood swings. These are the vitamins that support the immune system by reducing the impact of stress on one's life.

Vitamin B1 (thiamine) is a B-complex vitamin that's helpful for cell respiration, metabolism, heart health, and proper growth of the body.

Vitamin B2 (riboflavin) is used by the body to metabolize proteins and lipids; supply oxygen to cells; and repair the skin and nails. It is especially needed during stressful times.

Vitamin B3 (niacin) is a nutrient that stimulates circulation. It aids memory function, releases histamines, and helps hyperactivity. It is an excellent vitamin for the nerves. It is essential for brain metabolism. It reduces tension, fatigue, depression, and insomnia.

Vitamin B5 (pantothenic acid) protects against respiratory infections and is a natural tranquilizer.

Vitamin B6 (pyridoxine) is used in hormone and antibody production, in the synthesis of DNA and RNA, and in the metabolism of fat, protein, and carbohydrates. It is nature's diuretic and is very useful in menstruation for the water gained at this time. It is excellent for insomnia.

Vitamin B12 is a nutrient that increases the body's resistance to infection. A person especially needs this vitamin when fatigued. It helps form red blood cells, and to prevent constipation.

Biotin is used for the proper functioning of skin, nerves, bone marrow, and reproductive glands. It helps metabolize carbohydrates and protein.

Choline vitamins help keep the nerve coverings (myelin) healthy, aid in the production of acetylcholine (a neurotransmitter), and help the body utilize fat and cholesterol.

Folic acid is used for red-blood-cell formation and the synthesis of inositol. It works with choline and is vital for nourishment of the brain. It has been shown to help reduce fat in the liver.

PABA (para-aminobenzoic acid) protects the body against free radicals and is part of the folic acid molecule.

In Dr. Earl Mindell's *Vitamin Bible*, he points out that, "vitamins cannot replace food," and that vitamins cannot be assimilated without ingesting food. He says that vitamins are not pep pills and have no caloric or energy value of their own. They are not substitutes for protein of any other nutrients such as mineral, fats, carbohydrates, or water. He emphasizes that **"we cannot take vitamins, stop eating, and expect to be healthy."**

MINERALS

Calcium: Vitamin D and calcium work together to keep your blood's calcium level normal. You also need vitamin D to help your bones hold onto their calcium. For the best protection against osteoporosis, try to get about 200 IU of vitamin D daily. The dynamic duo has a sidekick: magnesium. Magnesium helps you absorb calcium and use vitamin D properly.

Chromium: Although only needed by the body in small amounts, this mineral is critical in fighting germs and foreign bodies. It is relatively easy to get at least 50 mcg of chromium a day from your food. Apples, broccoli, barley, corn, beef, eggs, nuts, mushrooms, oysters, rhubarb, tomatoes, and sweet potatoes are all good sources. Most good daily multi supplements also have some chromium in them.

Iodine: This mineral helps the thyroid gland produce the hormone thyroxin. It also helps absorb vitamin A. Lack of this nutrient can cause loss of interest and can produce a tendency toward obesity. The thyroid hormones play a big role in your growth, cell reproduction, nerve functions, and how your cells use oxygen. Some foods that contain iodine are dulse, kelp, agar, carrots, blueberries, cucumbers, eggplant, fish, fish roe, garlic, kale, and leaf lettuce.

Magnesium: When a person is deficient in this mineral, she can experience a personality change. Magnesium produces properdin, a blood protein that fights invading viruses and bacteria. It is destroyed by alcohol, diuretics, white sugar, white flour, and high amounts of protein. This mineral works on the bowels, muscles, and nerves. Some foods that contain magnesium are turnip greens, black walnuts, goat's milk, tofu, apricots, apples, green peppers, oats, prunes, figs, dulse, and lentils.

Manganese: It activates enzymes that work with vitamin C. As a team, they fight toxins and free radicals. It also stimulates the release of histamine, which protects the immune system. It is destroyed by high meat intake, excess phosphorus, and calcium, which act on the brain and nerves. Some foods that contain manganese are almonds, apples, apricots, green beans, blackberries, butternuts, celery, walnuts, oats, olives, and parsley.

Selenium: This is a very important trace mineral. It manifests anti-cancer effects. Cancer rates are lowest in regions with selenium-rich soil. It inhibits breast, skin, liver, and colon cancer. Selenium is lost in food processing. Brown rice has fifteen times the selenium content of white rice. Whole-wheat bread contains twice as much as white bread. Selenium and vitamin E work together to protect the body's cells. Selenium may also help protect you against heart disease. It also helps your immune system work effectively and helps remove heavy metals, such as lead, from your body.

Zinc: This is very important for your immune system. It strengthens the thymus gland, which is responsible for the production of T-lymphocytes. This mineral is healing to the mucus membranes.

10 HELPFUL SUGGESTIONS FOR EATING

In her book *Heal Yourself with Natural Foods*, Dr. Nancy Appleton has the following suggestions for eating:

1. Chew each mouthful of food at least 20–28 times.
2. Only drink liquid when there is no food in your mouth, so that you don't swallow the food undigested.
3. Drink most of your liquid between meals.
4. Consume only portions you feel you can safely digest.
5. When you are emotionally upset or disturbed, eat smaller portions and chew more thoroughly.
6. Undercook rather than overcook your food. This means lightly steam your vegetables and cook beans and proteins at low temperatures.
7. Boil, bake, steam, stir fry, or slow cook your food, rather than broil or fry it.
8. The more raw food you eat, the better.
9. Eat frequent, small meals, rather than fewer, large meals.
10. Examine each meal and snack from the viewpoint of, "Does any part of this meal upset my body chemistry and promote the disease process?"

DETOXIFICATION

The non-organic food we consume is sprayed with pesticides, our seafood is contaminated with mercury, we are ingesting chemicals from the air (vehicles, factory fumes), our drinking water is contaminated, and we are ingesting more synthetic prescriptions and over-the-counter medications. Our cells and tissues are bombarded with toxins, giving rise to many chronic diseases. Therefore, to keep our cells and tissues clean, we need to detoxify our systems.

We should understand why it is necessary to eat properly, take the right supplements, and get the proper amount of sleep and exercise. We have to realize that our lifestyle — the way we eat, sleep, and play — affects our blood and digestive system.

CONSTIPATION

In one of my first iridology classes, I was taught that the colon could be the graveyard of the body. To me, this means that all waste matter passes through the large intestines, and if this waste is not eliminated within a reasonable time, it lodges in the colon and can remain there, like something dead.

Our bodies are like chemical factories, constantly working and producing waste. Many natural medicine practitioners say you should have at least two bowel movements daily if you are eating and drinking properly. "In a healthy body, waste travels through the digestive tract in a predictable, regular cycle, usually taking six to twenty-four hours to pass. However, sometimes the passage of this waste material is too slow and the result is called constipation." The medical advisor states that "constipation is passing hard or infrequent stools or straining to have a bowel movement." In his book, *Solve your Skin Problems*, Dr. Patrick Holford, states that "the health of the colon can have far-reaching effects on the rest; acne is no exception to this. In fact, naturopathic doctors, earlier this century considered acne to be the result of a build-up of toxins in the colon. One study showed that half the people with severe acne had higher-than-normal levels of bowel toxins in their blood streams. This usually happens when the bowels are not emptied regularly because of a sluggish digestive system and constipation."

Constipation is the number-one digestive disorder in the United States.

SYMPTOMS OF CONSTIPATION

- Difficulty passing stools.
- Decreased frequency passing stools.
- Bloated, tender abdomen.
- Loss of appetite.
- Flatulence.
- Malaise and lack of energy.

HOW DOES FIBRE WORK?

"Scientifically speaking, fibre consists of complex carbohydrate molecules. They are found only in plant food, such as whole grains, fruits, vegetables, beans, nuts, and seeds. Unlike fats, which get quickly sopped up in the small intestine, the complex, bulky carbohydrate molecule in fibre can't be absorbed at all. Our digestive system lacks the enzymes to break it down. As far as your small intestine is concerned, these fibrous foods are utterly worthless, so the small intestine quickly passes them on to the large intestine. The large intestine can't do much with the fibre, either. The bulky fibre retains lots of water and causes the intestine to feel full quickly; therefore, it passes through the intestine more quickly."

FOODS TO AVOID

Fried food or food high in saturated fat. Fat moves very slowly in the digestive tract.

Mucus-forming foods, such as all dairy products, fried and processed foods, refined flour and chocolate.

Caffeine and alcohol. These foods are dehydrating to the digestive system.

CLEANSING DIETS TO REVITALIZE ALL ORGANS

Cleansing diets are really very simple. They range from the simplest use of water (for 24 hours) to a juice fast (for 24 hours). Another method is to eat nothing but fresh fruits for a day. This type of diet helps the cells lose some of their poison into the intestinal tract, where it is filtered out by the kidneys and bowels.

VEGETARIAN DIET

More studies are emerging to show that it is very beneficial to eat lots of vegetables and fruits, and to cut down on animal products.

"Even the government has endorsed the healthfulness of a vegetarian diet, for the first time, in a new set of nutritional guidelines."

WHY A VEGETARIAN DIET?

A plant-based diet is linked not only to lower rates of heart disease and stroke, but also to significantly lower rates of the most common cancers. These include colon and lung cancers; breast cancer and ovarian cancer in women; and prostate cancer in men.

Low-fat vegetarian diets may also reduce the incidence of osteoporosis, adult-onset diabetes, hypertension, obesity, and many other illnesses.

In contrast, a meat-based diet is high in saturated fat, which your body converts to cholesterol. It's also high in iron, an oxidant that oxidizes cholesterol and can clog your arteries.

Iron also causes the formation of free radicals, which promote cancer and aging. A meat-based diet is low in the antioxidants that help prevent this from happening.

There is no cholesterol in a plant-based diet and, with few exceptions (avocados, seeds, nuts, and oils), a plant-based diet is low in total and saturated fat.

A plant-based diet is also low in oxidants like iron (it has enough iron without having too much), and high in antioxidants like beta-carotene, and Vitamins A, C, and E.

Meat contains virtually no dietary fibre, which is high in a plant-based diet.

During the past few years, scientists have discovered and documented new classes of chemicals that help prevent illness and slow the aging process. These include bioflavonoids, carotenoids, phytochemicals and other substances.

These substances are high in a plant-based diet. In other words, there are more reasons to eat a plant-based diet. The major reason for changing your diet and lifestyle, however, is not just to live longer or reduce the risk of illness and heart problems later on, but to improve your quality of life *right now*.

It has been proven that "vegetarians have much lower rates of hypertension, heart disease, cancer, diabetes, gallstones, and obesity compared to meat eaters."

TYPICAL DIET

Testimonials from hundreds of grateful participants have filled the book *Reversing Disease with Fork and Knife*. Using Dr. Diehl's CHIP program, this dietary program is one good way of taking responsibility for your own health. Winston Churchill once stated, "We are victims of the curse of plenty." Dr. Diehl points out that "the diseases that we are seeing today in our society are unknown in countries whose diets are much simpler and plant-food centred." These diseases were rare in most societies until the turn of the 20th century. "Today's bitter harvest of our affluent lifestyle is represented by heart disease, cancer, stroke, and diabetes." (CHIP program)

Many studies have cited ten causes of death related to poor nutrition, namely:

- heart disease;

- cancer;
- cardiovascular disease;
- accidents;
- pulmonary disease;
- pneumonia;
- diabetes;
- suicide;
- liver disease;
- atherosclerosis.

The provision and adaptation of a good and well-balanced diet will set a good and lasting example for your family about the importance of establishing and maintaining an association between good nutrition and the restoration and maintenance of good health. Your diet will have to be individualized, to suit who you are and what conditions ail you.

THE IMPORTANCE OF PHYSICAL ACTIVITY

According to information gathered from Canada's Physical Activity Guide, "We need to be active to be healthy. Our modern-day lifestyle and all the conveniences we've become used to have made us sedentary — and that's dangerous for our health. Sitting around in front of the TV or the computer, riding in the car for even a short trip to the store and using elevators instead of stairs or ramps all contribute to our inactivity. Physical inactivity is as dangerous as smoking!"

Scientists recommend an accumulated 60 minutes of physical activity every day to stay healthy or improve your health. Physical activity can be built into our daily routine. No matter your age, it is never too late to start building strength, adding to your endurance, and eating right.

If you exercise even as little as fifteen minutes a day, the germ-fighting white blood cells of your body will increase. Being active is much easier than most people think. The hardest part of exercising is to actually start.

Once you start, you can gradually build on your daily routine. A little exercise daily is better than a lot on the weekends.

The lymphatic system responds to the stimulation of exercise when using the rebounder (mini-trampoline). It is best if you use it for short periods several times daily. As a result of this daily program, deeper breathing and exhaling will come naturally. This will increase oxygen in the blood and brain. It will also increase the circulation of blood and lymphatic fluid, thus protecting the immune system. Exercise helps minimize stress and its detrimental effects on the body.

The benefits of regular exercise, as outlined in Canada's Physical Activity Guide, include the following:

- better health;
- improved fitness;
- better posture and balance;
- better self-esteem;
- weight control;
- stronger muscles and bones;
- more energy;
- relaxation and reduced stress;
- continued independence;
- a longer life.

Health risks for inactivity include the following:

- premature death;
- heart disease;
- obesity;
- high blood pressure;
- adult-onset diabetes;
- osteoporosis;
- stroke;

- depression;
- colon cancer.

The Canadian Physical Activity Guide has set out the following recommendations:

- For endurance activities, begin with light activities and progress to moderate and vigorous activities. (This will prevent or minimize any muscle soreness you might experience when you start out.)
- Use comfortable footwear that provides good cushioning and support.
- Wear comfortable clothing that suits your activity and the weather.
- Wear safety gear approved by the Canadian Standard Association (CSA), whenever appropriate (e.g., a helmet for cycling and in-line skating, along with knee, elbow, and wrist protectors and protective eye goggles for squash.

DEEP BREATHING EXERCISES

Since breathing is something we can control and regulate, it is a useful tool for achieving a relaxed and clear state of mind. E. Bourne, adapted from The Anxiety and Phobia workbook, states, "When we are tense we breathe shallowly and rapidly. When relaxed, you breathe more fully and more deeply, from the abdomen. By using deep abdominal breathing, you stimulate the relaxation response of our bodies, promoting calmness. Additionally, attending to your breath will help you connect your mind to your body."

These exercises are excellent for strengthening lung tissues and increasing lung capacity. Breathing exercises are most beneficial when done out of doors, particularly early in the morning, around sunrise. This is the time of day when the trees release the most oxygen into the air so there is more life force in the air.

For added benefit, focus your thoughts on a particular quality that you wish to develop (kindness, generosity, purity, harmony, etc.) during inhalation. While exhaling, you might try focusing your thoughts on releasing something undesirable (anger, jealousy, tension, etc.).

Of course, it is better not to do deep-breathing exercises in areas where there is a lot of traffic congestion or other forms of air pollution. These exercises will slowly build up your lung capacity and help cleanse the lymphatic system, thus improving your immunities. As well, they are calming and rejuvenating. If your lungs were congested, practicing these exercises may cause you to experience one or two colds, as the mucus congestion is eliminated. Do not try to repress the body's effort to rid it of toxins and waste. This is the only way for it to come out. It is also important to sleep with the window open, even in cold weather, to allow for circulation of fresh air while sleeping.

While walking...

> **Inhale for the count of four paces.**
> **Hold for the count of four paces.**
> **Exhale for the count of eight paces.**
> **Hold again for the count of four paces.**

Keep to the same ratio (inhale one, hold one, exhale two, hold one) and try to build up to seven or more paces for inhalation

While Relaxing...

You can do these exercises sitting, standing or lying down. Try to breathe from the stomach, using your diaphragm instead of from the top of your chest. You can practice this by putting your hand on your navel while breathing. Your hand should move out with the inhalation and back with the exhalation. The shoulder should not rise.

Inhale four seconds.
Hold sixteen seconds.
Exhale eight seconds.

HOW MUCH AND WHAT KIND OF EXERCISE?

Experts suggest 30 minutes or more at least three times per week.

Brisk walking or any type of aerobic activity that increases cardio-vascular fitness is beneficial, such as learning a new dance, practicing tai chi, or taking up a new sport (physical activity that challenges the brain). This may be because learning a new skill activates new patterns of brain activity, and may literally build new synaptic connections in areas of the brain that correspond with the learned skill. A social activity, like dancing or group exercise, may also be especially beneficial because it combines social interaction with physical activity. **The important thing is to do something. Any type of activity is better than being sedentary.**

WHAT EXERCISE DOES TO THE BRAIN

- Accumulating evidence from neuroscience research is shedding new light on the basic question of how exercise changes the brain.
- Exercise reduces grey matter loss. Highly fit people also show less degrees in grey matter in the cortex than are normally seen with aging, which may suggest exercise's protective effect against nerve cell death.
- Exercise promotes neurogenesis (increase in the generation and survival of new neurons). Laboratory animals that are allowed to run freely on an exercise wheel show an increase in the neuron in the hippocampus (a brain structure involved in memory formation).
- Exercise strengthens neural connections. In laboratory animals, running increases the number and density of nerve connections

(synapses), physically changing the structure of these nerve-signal pathways to make them more efficient at transmitting nerve signals.

- Exercise enhances blood flow. The brain is the most energy-hungry organ in the body. To function optimally, it needs lots of oxygen and glucose, provided by the blood that circulates into the brain via arteries and capillaries. Exercise increases the density and size of the brain capillaries, which in turn increases blood flow to the brain. This may, in turn, help support the survival of new neurons in the brain area, such as the hippocampus, which is involved in memory formation and may facilitate faster firing of neurons. "Just by moving your feet, you are literally building the structure of the brain."

CONTROL YOUR NUMBERS

"There is overwhelming evidence that the same lifestyle and dietary factors that contribute to heart disease also increase the risk of Alzheimer's disease and age-related cognitive decline. Therefore, managing your numbers — cholesterol, blood pressure, blood sugar, and weight — has become *a rallying cry for brain-health advocates.*"

Sam Gandy, a scientific advisor to the Alzheimer's Association, says, "there are multiple reasons why you should pay attention to these central problems you might have and get control of them." He continues, "many factors that are good for your heart turn out to be good for your brain, as well."

Obesity might be the biggest threat to longevity. Excessive weight is associated with vascular disease. A study of 1,449 Finns with body masses of more than 30 found an associated risk for dementia that was twice that of folks with lower body masses. People with high levels of cholesterol and blood pressure had a risk that was six times higher.

CHECKLIST FOR BRAIN HEALTHY LIFESTYLE

Do

- Exercise your body regularly and get involved in physical activity and leisure pursuits.
- Keep your mind exercised. Engage in active learning throughout life and pursue new experiences.
- Stay socially engaged with friends, family, and community groups.
- Take steps to manage stress.
- Eat a brain-healthy, balanced diet rich in omega-3 fatty acids, and consider taking a multivitamin supplement that includes antioxidants and folate.
- Eat a variety of colourful, cruciferous, and leafy green vegetables (broccoli, cauliflower, green lettuce, and spinach).
- Cut extra calories. The key to keeping the brain in top form may be a low-calorie diet. The older you get, the more your brain cells are damaged by inflammation and oxidation, two major risk factors for Alzheimer's. The cells also have a harder time being repaired. A study of mice showed that a low-calorie diet might have a great effect on brain aging. When scientists compared the brain cells of senior mice fed a low-calorie diet to those of similar mice on a traditional diet, they found a remarkable difference. The brain cells of the low-calorie mice continued to function as if they were still young.
- Antioxidants — vitamins C, E, and beta carotene — reduce oxidative damage to cells from free radicals.

Common Foods High in Antioxidants

Fruits: Prunes, raisins, blueberries, blackberries, strawberries, raspberries, plums, oranges, red grapes, and cherries.

Vegetables: Kale, spinach, Brussels sprouts, alfalfa sprouts, broccoli florets, beets, red bell peppers, onions, corn, and eggplant.

- Mind your numbers: lose any extra pounds, lower your cholesterol if it is high, and keep blood glucose and blood pressure under control.
- Get adequate sleep.
- Get proper medical attention and treatment for any underlying health problems.

Don't

- Drink to excess, smoke, or use illicit drugs.
- Ignore sudden changes in mental status but don't be overly concerned about normal slips of memory or where you put your keys.
- Put off going to the doctor if you notice changes in your health, physically or mentally.
- Overlook the possibility of drug interactions that can affect mental functioning, especially if you were taking more than one prescription medication.
- Become isolated in your home.
- Think you're too old to take up something new.

ASPECTS OF SOCIAL WELLNESS

A well-adjusted person in our modern-day society is considered one who is able to associate or mix socially with other people. There are many factors that influence our social wellness. These include the following.

- Our religious background. Going to church or religious meetings with our parents where we meet other people with similar beliefs and interests.
- Institutions of learning. From our first day in kindergarten through grade school, middle school, high school and post-graduate studies, we meet and make friends with many people. Some of these we cherish as dear friends whose company we value and respect. When we can make and sustain a cordial relationship or friendship with another human being, I think we have mastered social wellness.

ASPECTS OF SPIRITUAL WELLNESS

As a citizen with a West Indian background, I can truly say I was born in the lap of deep spirituality. Speaking as a true Jamaican-born woman, I was taught to pray from a very young age. I was sent to Sunday school every Sunday and taught to revere God. I got saved at the early age of twelve. I asked God, the master and director of my life, for his holy spirit to live within my heart. I derive great blessings from reading the Bible and listening to gospel music and meditating on my Lord. I take pride in treating others the way that I would have them treat me. I know that God has no hands or feet in our physical world, so we who are called by his name should be our brother's keeper. These are some of the things I practice for my spiritual wellness:

- I try to read the Bible on a daily basis.
- I always take time for myself, especially at night before going to sleep. I lie quietly in bed and talk to my creator. I talk to him like I am talking to a dear friend. I try not to complain, but sometimes I ask him why certain things happen to me. He reveals his answers to me in his own time.
- I have received healing many times from my friend and creator.
- I try not to depend on my own wisdom, but to trust God for everything.
- I try not to judge other people.
- I try to listen to the voice of God at all times and I ask him to lead me in this fallen world. I ask him to hold my hand and to never let go, because if I hold his hand I may feel tired and let go.

This physical world is ruled by principalities and powers. Ephesians 6:12 says, "For we wrestle not against flesh and blood, but against principalities, against powers, against rulers of the darkness of this world, against spiritual wickedness in high places."

Ephesians 5:13 says, "Wherefore take unto you the whole armour of God, that ye may be able to withstand in the evil day, and having done all, to stand." (Please read the remainder of this chapter in Ephesians and you will appreciate the full meaning of spiritual wellness.)

To be spiritual in today's society, you must seek God's guidance each day, because principalities and powers (evil leaders making evil laws) have escalated their games, and this will only harm our children and bring damnation to our world.

Here are some tips and suggestions to help improve your spiritual health:

ASSESSING YOUR SPIRITUAL WELLNESS

- Where are you in your spiritual life?
- Take a moment to reflect…. Do you feel a sense of worth, hope, purpose, commitment, and peace?
- Do you have a positive outlook on life or do you experience feelings of emptiness, anxiety, hopelessness, apathy, or conflict?

These may be signs of spiritual poverty in your life and may be the reason for unhappiness or dissatisfaction. Please go through this simple exercise by asking yourself these questions. It may help to make you more spiritually grounded.

SPIRITUAL SUPPORT IN PRAYER

Twelve Gallup polls over the last 35 years have found that most Americans believe in the power of prayer to heal, and medical experts are coming to that same conclusion. Researchers actually did a scientific study to find out whether people cope with life stresses (like major illness) better if they have a strong faith and pray regularly. The conclusion? Yes, they cope better. The word *prayer* comes from the Latin word *precarious*, which means "obtained by begging, to entreat." Prayer is rooted in the belief that there is a power greater than oneself that can influence one's life. It is the act of raising hearts and minds to God or a higher power.

Prayer is comforting and you can do it by yourself. Don't worry about anything; instead, pray about everything. Tell God what you need, and thank him for all he has done.

Prayer is important in a health-care context simply because it is used so widely. According to Dr. Wayne Jonas, "Surveys indicate that nearly 90% of patients with serious illness will engage in prayer for the alleviation of their suffering or disease." Among all forms of complementary medicine, prayer is the single most widely practiced healing modality. Research conducted by Dr. Christine Puchalski, director of the George Washington Institute for Spirituality and Health, says prayer is the second-most common method of pain management (after oral pain management), and the most non-drug method for managing pain.

HOW PRAYER IMPROVES HEALTH

- *The relaxation response.* Prayer elicits the relaxation response, which lowers blood pressure and relieves stress.
- *The opportunity to unload inner conflict.* There is much to be gained by pouring out your soul to your creator without worry about being criticized or judged.
- *Peace.* After pouring your soul to God, you will feel his divine peace flowing in your heart.
- *The placebo response.* Prayer can enhance a person's hope and expectations and that, in turn, can positively impact health.
- *A healing presence.* Prayer can bring a sense of a spiritual or loving presence and alignment with God, or immersion into a closeness with your creator.
- *Positive feelings.* Prayer can elicit feelings of gratitude, compassion, forgiveness, and hope, all of which are associated with healing and wellness.
- *Mind-body-spirit connection.* When prayer uplifts or calms, it inhibits the release of cortisol and other hormones, thus reducing the negative impact on the immune system and promoting healing.

ASPECTS OF ENVIRONMENTAL WELLNESS

Although some environmental concerns are beyond our control, there are things that can be done to promote a healthier earth. Many of us are not aware that our surroundings play a very important role in our lives.

Light: Light plays an important role in balancing mental health. During the winter when the sun is sometimes obscured, many people suffer from winter blahs or some form of depression. Light therapy is very helpful.

Temperature: Too much heat or cold can also be a problem. Getting too chilly can suppress the immune system and leave you susceptible to cold and infections.

Dental fillings: The mercury in a filling can play a role in disease in the mouth. Some of the oral health problems in play are foul breath, bleeding gums, grinding teeth, metallic taste, and periodontal disease.

Technology: Technology is a double-edged sword. Don't abuse it. Television emits low-grade ionized radiation. Sit at least ten feet away while watching TV. Microwave cooking does the same thing and, in addition, seems to change the chemical molecular structure of food. When its molecular structure is changed, it's more difficult to digest because we do not have the enzymes to digest food that has been restructured. According to Dr. Appleton, to minimize the possible dangerous exposure to electromagnetic fields, stay several feet from appliances that produce such fields. She suggests the recommended distances for the following appliances:

- Fans: two to three feet.
- Electric clocks: three to four feet.
- Computers: three to four feet.
- Copying machines, laser printers, fax machines: five feet.

- Electric blankets also produce an electric field that may increase the risk of breast cancer. Turn on the blanket before you retire, but turn it off before you get into bed.

Aluminum cookware has no place in the kitchen. Research shows that when water in aluminum cookware is heated to only 88 degrees (water boils at 212 degrees), there is a 74-fold increase in aluminum in the water. That is 30 times more than the recommended water quality limit. There is some evidence that links excessive aluminum with Alzheimer's disease and other conditions.

Use free or non-toxic paint. New carpets can also cause problems. If you redecorate, you should leave your home for about a week so that the paint and carpets can discharge their chemically filled fumes. Leave as many windows open as possible.

Additive alert:

"You are what you eat," the sage said. Today, we eat not only food but a lot of chemicals added to food to give it flavour or colour, or to keep it fresh and free from bugs and diseases.

ASPECTS OF OCCUPATIONAL WELLNESS

Occupational/vocational wellness involves preparing and making use of your gifts, skills, and talents in order to gain purpose, happiness, and enrichment in your life. The development of occupational satisfaction and wellness is related to your attitude about your work. Achieving optimal occupational wellness allows you to maintain a positive attitude and experience satisfaction/pleasure in your employment.

The occupationally well individual contributes his/her skills/talents to work that is meaningful and rewarding. Values are expressed through involvement in activities that are personally rewarding for you and make a contribution to the well-being of the community at large. Occupational wellness means successfully integrating a commitment to your occupation into a total lifestyle that is satisfying and rewarding.

This may involve the actual work you do, the roles that you play, and/or the responsibilities that you have as a full-time parent or student. Being occupationally well means seeking opportunities to grow professionally and being fulfilled in your job, whatever it may be.

Tips and suggestions for optimal occupational wellness include the following:

- Explore a variety of career options.
- Create a vision for your future.
- Choose a career that suits your personality, interests, and talents.
- Visit a career planning/placement office and use the available resources.
- Be open to change and learning new skills.

Manage your time

Avoid multitasking

Accept your fear

Avoiding Stress

Seek support from others

Talk to someone

Think positively

Try relaxation techniques

STRESS AND WELLNESS

As long as we can cope with any stressful situation, we should not think it is so bad. It can be beneficial in that it challenges and motivates us to accomplish great things.

Stress can be bad when we are no longer able to cope. It is during this period that stress can interfere with our wellness/health.

FIGHT-OR-FLIGHT RESPONSE

The way we respond to problems in our lives may also be a type of stress. When faced with a problem or threat, your body can activate resources to protect — to either run as fast as you can or stay and fight (the fight-or-flight response). This is our body's sympathetic nervous system reacting to a stressful situation. Large amounts of cortisol, adrenalin, and noradrenalin are produced. This triggers a higher heart rate, increased sweating, and alertness to protect us, if need be. When we are in a state of stress, our non-essential body functions are slowed and hormones are concentrated on rapid breathing, increased blood flow, alertness, and muscle use.

When we are stressed, the following happens:

- blood pressure rises;
- breathing becomes more rapid;
- the digestive system slows down;
- the heart rate increases;
- the immune system decreases;
- our muscles become tense;
- we do not sleep well.

How we respond to stress affects our health.

It is very important to realize that the interpretation of events and challenges in life may be the deciding factor to harm or heal you. A negative response to events can eventually have a negative effect on your health and happiness. In a study done at Pennsylvania State University, investigators found that *stress is not the problem, but how we react to stressors is.* It appears that how clients react to stress is a predictor of their health, a decade later, regardless of their present health and stressors.

HOW TO DEAL WITH MODERN-DAY STRESS

- The first thing I always ask my clients is to identify what the cause of their stress is.
- When they do, they will be able to work through the stressors.
- I always encourage journaling. It helps the client to express her feelings through writing. She will then express her fears and insecurities.
- Clients are encouraged to take responsibility for their own health by trying to eat properly, doing some exercise (even forcing oneself to exercise, if need be), taking time to relax by listening to soothing music.

BELIEVE IN YOURSELF

According to Shad Helmstetter, "Your success or failure in anything large or small will depend on your programming: what you accept from others and what you say when you talk to yourself. Remember, what you put in, you get out (it does not matter if you believe it or not). The brain simply believes what you tell it (it does not care whether it is right or wrong). **What you think you will become."**

Here are a few tips on how to believe in yourself:

- Keep your priorities straight.
- Take responsibility for yourself.
- Create your own future.

- Focus on what you want.
- Learn to visualize the outcome of your destiny.
- Think positively.
- Set specific goals and review them often.

SPECIAL NOTE ON SLEEP/REST

"Sleep is absolutely essential to both body and mind. Impaired sleep, altered sleep patterns, and sleep deprivation wreck havoc on mental and physical functions. Many health conditions — particularly depression, chronic fatigue syndrome, and fibromyalgia — are [at least] partially related to sleep deprivation or disturbed sleep" (*Natural Medicine*).

Physiologically, sleep is a complex process of restoration and renewal for the body. Scientists still do not know a definitive explanation as to why humans have a need for sleep. We do know that sleep is not a passive switching-off of bodily functions; sleep is believed to be important and has many good benefits.

RECOMMENDATIONS TO HELP YOU SLEEP

- In the evening, eat bananas, dates, figs, milk, and whole-grain crackers. These food are high in tryptophan, which promotes sleep.
- Do not eat large meals within two hours of bedtime.
- Avoid caffeine, alcohol, and nicotine for four to six hours before bedtime.
- Go to bed only when you are sleepy.
- Do not stay in bed if you are not sleepy.
- Sleep in a dark, quiet room with a comfortable temperature.
- Do not exercise within two hours of bedtime.

CHAPTER SIX

COMMON AILMENTS: KNOW YOUR RISK FACTORS

There are many factors that might increase your risk for the following diseases. It is very important that you discuss genetic illness or predispositions with your parents, grandparents, or caregivers, especially in relation to the diseases listed below:

- Diabetes
- Heart Disease
- High Blood Pressure
- High Cholesterol
- Cancers
- Obesity
- Prostate Problem
- Osteoporosis

SPECIAL NOTES ON SOME VERY COMMON AILMENTS

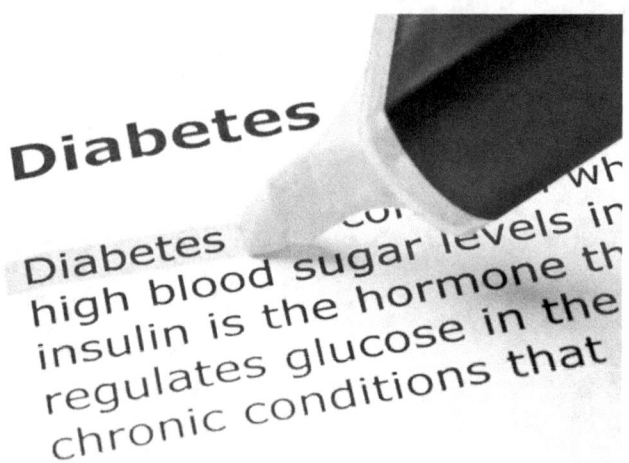

DIABETES

Diabetes is a metabolic disorder in which the body's ability to manufacture insulin is diminished. Insulin is a crucial hormone that enables blood sugar to enter the body's cells, to be used for energy. The elevated level of glucose in the bloodstream damages the cells. Since cells are the basic unit of life, diabetes ultimately affects the entire body.

There are two types of diabetes, namely:

Type 1 diabetes. This was once known as juvenile onset diabetes because most (but not all) of the cases develop in childhood. This type is characterized by a destruction of the cells in the pancreas that produced insulin.

Type 2 diabetes. In this form of the disease, the body does produce insulin, but the amount may be diminished and people's bodies are unable to use it properly. The form of the disease typically occurs in people over the age of forty-five who have other risk factors.

HOW TO REDUCE THE RISK FOR DIABETES:

Some experts estimate that up to 80% of diabetes diagnoses can be prevented by lifestyle changes, primarily losing weight and exercising. Furthermore, if you successfully stave off developing diabetes, you've dramatically lowered your risk for heart disease and stroke, two major killers.

You can greatly reduce your risk of getting diabetes by:

- slimming down;
- adopting healthy eating habits;
- exercising

Although it is seldom recognized, diabetes is one of the greatest and most preventable health problems today. If you are at risk of developing diabetes, change your lifestyle. Eat healthily and keep moving.

HEART DISEASE

Heart disease is one of the biggest killers of women, yet many women continue to be misdiagnosed and ignored. Actually an umbrella term that encompasses many different types of malaise, heart disease includes the following:

- congestive heart failure;
- congenital heart defects;
- malfunctioning heart valves;
- coronary heart disease, also called atherosclerosis (the disease process that narrows the heart's coronary arteries and results in heart attacks);
- smoking;
- high blood pressure;
- diabetes;
- high cholesterol.

Whatever the reason, tissues try to heal themselves. In heart disease, a combination of overgrown tissue, immune cells, and fat known as plaque accumulates. This disease process is known as atherosclerosis. As it does, beneath the arteries' lining, the artery becomes narrower and narrower. If the blood supply were squeezed off or a clot forms and blocks it, the result is a heart attack.

HOW TO REDUCE THE RISK OF A HEART ATTACK:

- Do not smoke.
- Lose weight.
- Start exercising.
- Consider aspirin (if you are middle aged or have a high risk for heart attacks, speak to your doctor about daily aspirin to prevent blood clots).
- Reduce your stress.

HEART ATTACK WARNING SIGNS

- Sudden chest pain that intensifies over a minute or two.
- Pain in the centre of the chest that's not relieved by rest or changing position.
- Pain lasting at least 20 minutes.
- The pain ranges from mild to severe and usually feels like tightness or heaviness.
- The pain radiates to your jaw, your back, or down your left arm.
- You experience nausea, shortness of breath, or a sense of impending doom.

Do not ignore the warning signs of a heart attack. If you think you are having a heart attack, do not drive yourself to the hospital. When you reach the emergency room, state that you believe you are having a heart attack, and describe your symptoms as specifically as possible.

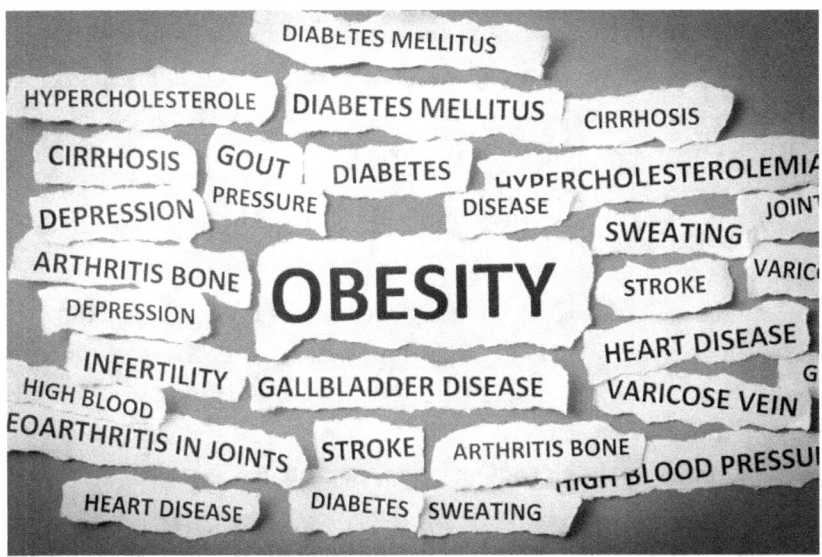

OBESITY

One of our biggest modern-day plagues is obesity. Obesity is defined as being more than 20% over the ideal weight. It is estimated that more than 80 million Americans are overweight. Symptoms of obesity include having excessive fat on your body, shortness of breath, and palpitations of the heart on exertion. (*Back to Eden*). Our Western diet is killing us. Poor eating habits and eating the wrong type of food have led us to an epidemic of obesity in North America. "Eating too much and eating too frequently produce a feverish state in the system and overtax the digestive organs." (*Back to Eden*) We are eating unhealthy foods and the storage of excess fat is a "sign that your cells may be receiving damaging communication from this unhealthy food, giving rise to obesity. Our poor diet is high in refined foods, high caloric foods, and snacking between meals. Our bodies are experiencing unregulated cell growth which we call obesity."

Effects of overeating:

- The blood becomes impure and diseases of various kinds occur such as different types of cancer, kidney disease, diabetes, gallstones, osteoarthritis, arteriosclerosis, high blood pressure, and strokes.
- Excessive acid produced in the body.
- The mucus lining of the stomach becomes congested.
- High levels of cholesterol and triglycerides in the blood.

"The modern way in which food is being served is very destructive. The meal is arranged so that the most highly tempting dishes — such as pastries, ice cream, etc. — are presented last. This encourages excessive eating. After having eaten enough, a person adds this extra rich food which becomes a burden and poison to the system."

When the stomach and intestines are already full of food, any additional food is forced to remain in the stomach. Over time, this food sours. When this happens, its poisons are absorbed into the bloodstream and, consequently, the whole system is affected. Overeating works the heart, stomach, liver, kidneys, and bowels much harder.

In order to lose weight, you must first decide if you really want to do so.

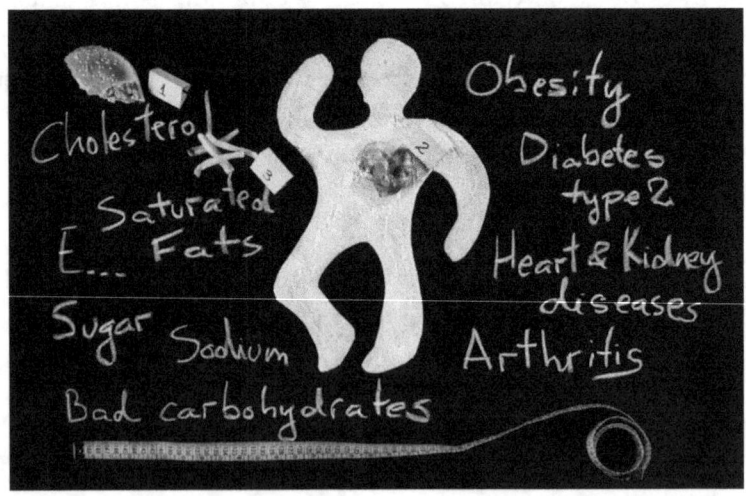

SUGGESTIONS TO HELP YOU LOSE WEIGHT

- Don't lose weight too rapidly. You should lose between one-half and two pounds each week.
- Don't eat snacks between meals.
- Eat a good nutritional breakfast (the most important meal of the day).
- Avoid foods that are high in calories.
- Eat fresh fruits instead of desserts.
- Leave the table while you are still a bit hungry. Don't have second servings.
- Cut down on fatty foods.
- Establish a regular exercise program and stick to it.
- Drink a glass of water immediately upon awaking (this will start cleaning the body).
- Drink eight glasses of water during the day (this will help flush toxins from your fat cells).
- Walk as much as possible. The body was made for walking. Research has shown that one hour of walking each day will change your body dramatically. Start slowly, maybe ten minutes daily, and gradually build up.
- Do not eat after six p.m. Do not use diet sodas or diet food.
- Do not eat from any fast food restaurants.
- Do not use any artificial sweeteners.
- Do not use any white sugar or flour. White sugar is very addictive, and white flour, when mixed, forms a paste that clogs up your digestive system, slowing down your metabolism.
- Do a liver cleanse. If you are overweight, your liver is definitely clogged.

Please take charge and do what you have to do to lose weight.

You will feel better and you will be healthier.

METABOLIC SYNDROME

WHY IS YOUR BELLY SO BIG?

As a young girl growing up in Jamaica, I always observed people, both men and women, with very *BIG bellies* or abdomens. I used to wonder why they had such big bellies, but there was no answer. I completed nursing school and did not learn anything about metabolic syndrome. I am very happy I did this research thesis because now I am getting a bird's-eye view as to the cause of this big belly dilemma. Travelling on the buses, walking the street, every other person that passes you by has a *big belly*.

According to a comprehensive article by AstraZeneca on metabolic syndrome, abdominal obesity — in other words, *big belly* — is an important component of metabolic syndrome.

This "big belly syndrome" is known by several names, including:

- abdominal obesity;
- belly fat;
- central obesity (clinically);
- metabolic syndrome;
- MetS;
- Syndrome X.

"Metabolic syndrome (MetS) or Syndrome X is a term recently created to group together carbohydrate and lipid anomalies associated with insulin resistance, hypertension, and intestinal obesity." (Alternative Medicine College of Canada)

The World Health Organization has recognized this condition since 1998 and American authorities have since 2001.

Metabolic syndrome has become a dominant pathology in our society, notably because of the frequency of the associated cardiovascular complications. It is a common pathology linked largely to our Western lifestyle, unbalanced diet, and sedentary lifestyle.

There are three great schools of thought on this modern-day plague. They are:

1. WHO, published in 1998 and amended in 1999.
2. American National Cholesterol Education Program (NCEP-ATP lll), published in 2001.
3. International Diabetes Federation, published in 2005.

The definitions given by these three all take into consideration an association of risk factors:

- hypertension;
- hypertriclyceridemia;
- a low level of HDH-cholesterol;
- android obesity (pear-shaped abdominal obesity);
- elevated blood sugar levels;
- insulin-resistance syndrome;
- dysmetabolic syndrome.

According to literature by the Alternative Medicine College of Canada, "metabolic syndrome can be explained by the inter-relation that exists between dysglycemia, the anomalies of lipid balance, and hypertension." The article continues, "This syndrome is characterized by insulin resistance linked to an abnormal production of cytokine by the fat cells. It results in a plasma excess of free fatty acids that exercise their toxicity particularly at the hepatic and muscular levels. Type 2 diabetes and the dyslipidemia that follows contribute, along with hypertension and hemostasis anomalies, to lesions of the vascular endothelium and to atheromatosis."

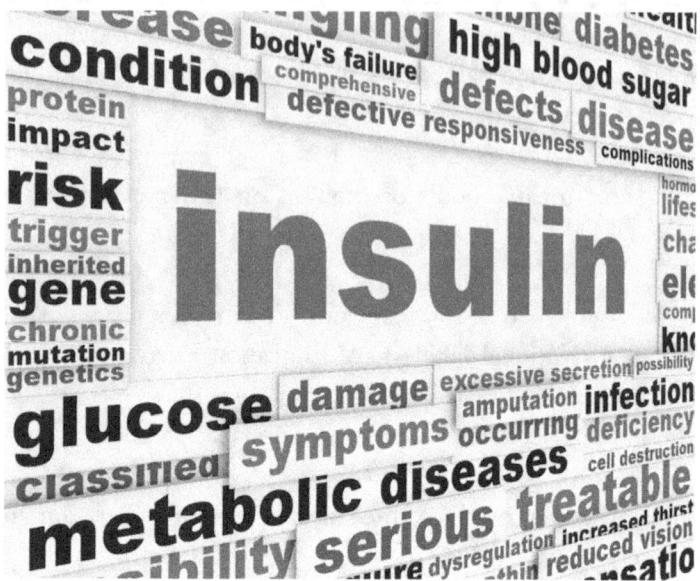

According to an article on Wikipedia, this syndrome also causes excessive abdominal fat around the stomach and abdomen. Abdominal obesity is not confined to the elderly and obese. It has been linked to Alzheimer's disease, as well as to other metabolic and vascular diseases.

CAUSE OF METABOLIC SYNDROME

According to studies done at Cleveland Clinic, "the exact cause of metabolic syndrome is not known. Many features of [the condition] are associated with insulin resistance. Insulin resistance means that the body does not use insulin efficiently to lower glucose and triglyceride levels. Insulin resistance is a combination of genetic and lifestyle factors."

A recent national health survey indicated that, "more than one in five North Americans has metabolic syndrome." The number of people with metabolic syndrome increases with age, affecting more than 40% of people in their 60s and 70s.

- Metabolic syndrome increases the risk of diabetes and cardiovascular disease.
- About one in four adults has metabolic syndrome.
- Incidences of metabolic syndrome increase with age.
- Metabolic syndrome increases heart-disease risk in women under the age of 65 with other risk factors.
- Men aged 35 to 65 have a higher prevalence of the major risk factors.
- The main causes are: obesity, physical inactivity, and genetic factors.
- The risk factors are easily measured and can be managed.

HIGH BLOOD PRESSURE (HYPERTENSION)

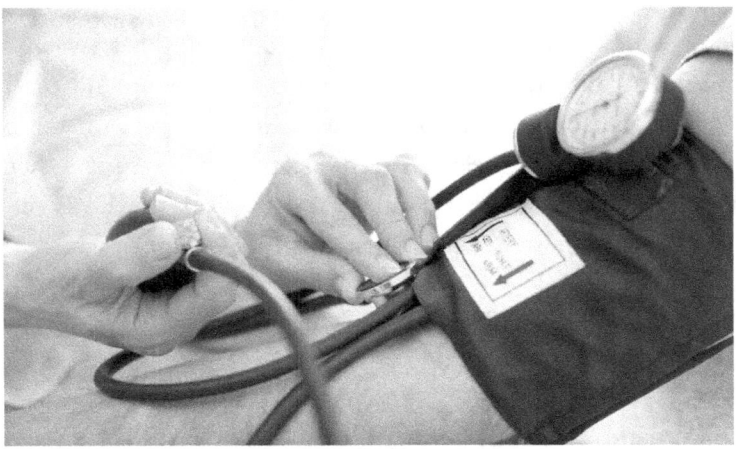

Blood pressure is the pressure of the blood against the walls of the blood vessels. The term usually refers to the pressure of the blood within the arteries, or arterial blood pressure. Blood pressure is determined by the following factors:

- The pumping action of the heart.
- The resistance to the flow of blood in the arterioles.
- The elasticity of the walls of the main arteries.

- The quantity of blood within the blood vessels.
- The viscosity or thickness of the blood.

There are actually two blood pressures with the blood vessels during one complete beat of the heart, a higher pressure during the contraction phase (systolic) and a lower pressure during the relaxation phase (diastolic).

High blood pressure usually creeps up with no warning or symptoms. Doctors call this disease a silent killer for good reason. It is the biggest risk factor for the above ailment, and also for erectile dysfunction and even blindness.

ZEROING IN ON THE SILENT KILLER: HIGH BLOOD PRESSURE

Blood pressure is the force exerted by the contracting heart against the blood vessels as it pumps blood through the vessels around the body. Every time your heart beats, blood exerts extra pressure on the blood vessels' walls . The first beat is called the systolic pressure. When the heart rests between beats, this is called the diastolic pressure. We get high blood pressure when we have a regularly high blood pressure reading.

Here is a quick guide to blood pressure numbers:

Blood Pressure Category	Systolic mmHg (Upper#)	Diastolic mmHg (Lower#)
Average	less than 120	less than 80
Prehypertension	120-139	80-89
Stage 1	140-159	90-99
Stage 2	160 or higher	100 or higher

In hypertension, the blood pressure is constantly higher than it should be, whether you are stressed or relaxed.

Ninety percent of people with high blood pressure have primary (essential) hypertension. Some of the contributing factors in high blood pressure are:

- Heredity
- Excessive weight
- Stress
- Lack of exercise
- High salt intake
- Alcohol consumption
- Smoking
- Age
- Excessive use of stimulants such as coffee and drug abuse.

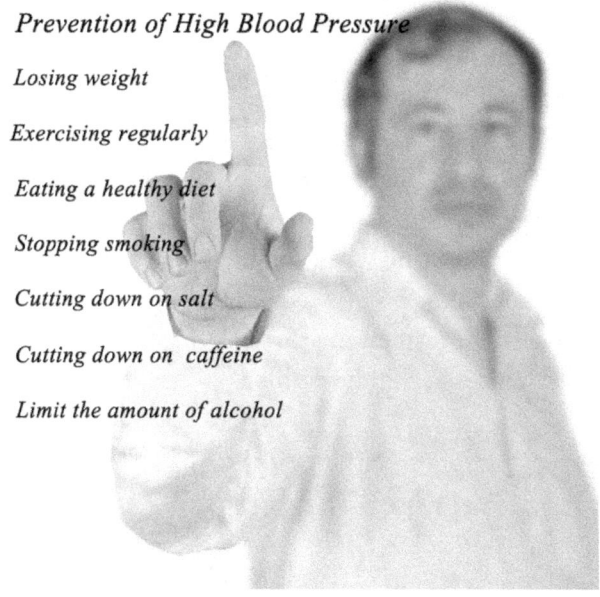

Prevention of High Blood Pressure

Losing weight

Exercising regularly

Eating a healthy diet

Stopping smoking

Cutting down on salt

Cutting down on caffeine

Limit the amount of alcohol

The other ten percent is the result of other ailments. This condition is called secondary hypertension. It can be caused by the blood vessels being chronically constricted or having lost their elasticity from a build-up of fatty plaque on their inside walls, a condition known as atherosclerosis. Arteriosclerosis and atherosclerosis are common precursors to hypertension. The narrowing and/or hardening of the arteries makes circulation of blood through the vessels difficult, giving rise to poor circulation and high blood pressure. Some of the contributing factors are:

- Kidney disease
- Thyroid problems
- Adrenal problems
- Sleep apnea.

SOME SIGNS OF POOR CIRCULATION:

- Arms and legs going to sleep.
- A sharp diagonal crease in your ear (heart-head connection).
- A short walk may cause aches and pains.
- A nagging cough.
- A whitish ring under the outer part of the cornea.
- A tingling sensation in your lips and fingers.
- Breathlessness on slight exertion or on lying down.
- Cold fingers and toes.
- Cramps in your hand when you write.
- Poor memory.
- Numbness or heaviness in arms or legs.
- Swollen ankles late in the evening.

RECOMMENDATIONS TO HELP WITH HIGH BLOOD PRESSURE

- Reduce your salt intake. Practice reading labels carefully and cut out foods that contain high sodium/salt and other additives such as MSG.
- Eat plenty of fruits and vegetables, including apples, bananas, grapefruits, prunes, raisins, green leafy vegetables, cabbage, melons, squash, and sweet potatoes

- Drink around eight glasses of distilled water daily.
- Use skinless chicken and fish, and get other protein from vegetable sources such as grains and legumes.
- Keep your weight down.
- Get regular mild to moderate exercise.
- Get adequate sleep.
- Avoid stress.
- Avoid chocolate, pickled foods and sour cream.
- Cayenne pepper and garlic are powerful foods that help in the control of high blood pressure.
- Quit smoking.
- Cut back on alcohol.
- Cut down on junk food.

SPECIAL NOTE ON CHOLESTEROL

The National Heart, Lung, and Blood Institute states, "High blood cholesterol is one of the major risk factors for heart disease. In fact, the higher your blood cholesterol, the greater your risk of developing heart disease or having a heart attack." Cholesterol causes heart disease when there is too much in the blood. This fat-like substance sticks to the walls of your arteries and, over time, this build-up causes "hardening of the arteries" so that the arteries become slowed down or blocked. This may cause chest pain or even a heart attack.

According to Statistics Canada, "Although cholesterol is essential for human health, a high level of cholesterol in the bloodstream can lead to damaged vessels and cardiovascular disease. Monitoring cholesterol, for the management of abnormal levels and the prevention of cardiovascular disease, is particularly important for males over 40 years of age, as well as menopausal females or females over 50 years of age. People with diabetes and atherosclerosis or people who have a risk factor such as smoking, abdominal obesity, hypertension, or a strong family history of hypertension, need to pay attention."

Cholesterol isn't all bad. It is a type of fat that's actually a nutrient. But as you've probably heard, there's good cholesterol and bad cholesterol. When we measure cholesterol and blood fats, we're really talking about three different numbers:

1. HDL
2. LDL
3. triglycerides

They combine to give you a lipid profile score, but the three individual scores are most important.

OSTEOPOROSIS

Osteoporosis is also called "the silent killer," because it steals strength from your skeleton. It has few warning signs until, suddenly, you break a bone. When you are young, your bones get longer and denser until you reach full height. During your growing period, your bone tissue is constantly being broken down and rebuilt. When a woman reaches her early 30s and a man his early 40s, their skeletons begin to lose bone faster than their bodies can replace it. Osteoporosis affects more women than men because the hormone estrogen plays a crucial role in the female body's ability to use dietary calcium to build new bone. When a woman approaches menopause, the reduction of the body's estrogen production deprives bone of the calcium needed. Twenty to thirty percent of bone loss in women occurs in the first five years after menopause.

The skeleton gradually thins as you age. If you have osteoporosis, this is a different story. By the time you are being diagnosed, your bones will already have lost significant density, making them fragile and easy to break, often spontaneously or after a very minor accident.

This is the slow, insidious loss of bone mass, a weakening of the bone structure that contributes to hip fractures, lower back pain, and, sometimes death. This degenerative disease begins slowly. For women, it is accelerated by menopause, and in men it sometimes starts after 65 years. The main symptoms of osteoporosis are loss of height due to compression of the weakened vertebrae. The other symptoms are cramps in the legs and feet; bone pain; extreme fatigue; excessive plaque on the teeth; and fracture of the hip, spine, wrist or other part of the skeleton. A patient rarely feels any pain until the fracture occurs. It is not really a matter of inadequate calcium intake but a problem of body-chemistry upset that does not allow the calcium to be properly utilized.

Other signs and symptoms of osteoporosis:

- Dowager's hump (a forward bending of the upper spine);
- Ricketts;
- Brittle or soft fingernails;
- Premature grey hair;
- Heart palpitation (calcium deficiency).

NATURAL ALTERNATIVES TO OSTEOPOROSIS DRUGS:

- Diet and lifestyle changes. A diet rich in inflammation-fighting foods such as vegetables, fruits, nuts, and seeds is useful. Omega-3-rich fish such as wild salmon and sardines, and lean poultry are recommended.
- Avoid a high-sodium diet. Research has shown that a high-salt (sodium) diet contributes to calcium loss. Avoid packaged foods because they are high in sodium.
- Fermented soy foods and protein powders have been shown to increase bone formation.
- Eat sea vegetables. A half cup of wakame contains 1,700 mg of calcium, a quarter cup of agar contains 1,000 mg of calcium, a half

cup of nori contains 600 mg of calcium, a quarter cup of kombu contains 500 mg of calcium.

- Eat sardines. Sardines with bones are not only a good source of omega-3 fatty acids, but of calcium, with 500 mg per half cup.
- Vitamin K is important for proper bone formation. This nutrient is abundant in dark green leafy vegetables, such as lettuce, spinach, and broccoli.
- Regular weight-bearing exercise is critical for proper bone formation and the stimulation of increased bone density. Walking, jogging, and stair climbing are good.
- Weightlifting twice per week to focus on various parts of the skeleton is wise.
- If you smoke, stop.
- Calcium has been shown to help prevent osteoporosis and it helps to slow bone loss. *Use a dosage of 500 to 600 mg of well-absorbed calcium complexes twice daily.* Men with prostate cancer should not take more than 500 mg of calcium, unless instructed by their doctor.
- Magnesium is thought to be just as important as calcium for bone density. It is involved in parathyroid hormone production and the activation of vitamin D, both of which influence calcium metabolism and absorption. Dosage is 250 mg to 350 mg twice daily.
- Vitamin D has become a superstar in nutrition in recent years. Its value for osteoporosis prevention and treatment has been upgraded to that of a critically important nutrient. Dosage is 1,000 to 2,000 IU daily with meals.
- Vitamin K is a key player in bone calcification. It is required for the bone-forming protein osteocalcin to function properly. Dosage of vitamin K is 45 mg daily. Typical dosage for those with osteoporosis is 500 mg to 2,000 mg. If you are on blood-thinning medication, consult your doctor before taking vitamin K.
- Potassium is an important mineral for bone metabolism. Take up to 1,200 mg (daily) of potassium citrate. If you have a kidney problem or are on potassium-sparing high-blood-pressure medication, consult your doctor before taking potassium.

- Ipriflavone is a copy of the soy isoflavone daidzein. Several studies have shown that, when combined with calcium, this supplement can increase bone density. It has also been shown to prevent osteoporosis when taken in combination with estrogen or vitamin D. Ipriflavone stimulates bone-building cells known as osteoblasts. Dosage is 600 mg daily.
- Essential fatty acids are often deficient in a North American diet. They work to reduce inflammation, a foundational cause of osteoporosis. A study in The Journal of Aging reported that a combination of fish oil and evening primrose oil, along with 600 mg of calcium, improved bone density in senior women. Dosage is 1,500 of EPA and DHA, combine,d daily, and 500 mg GLA daily. Do not use fish oil if you are on blood-thinning medication unless under the supervision of a doctor.
- Horny goat weed contains two plant estrogens, also found in soy, that combat osteoporosis. Dosage is to take a horny goat product daily (contains 60 mg of icariin). Do not take if you're taking any blood-thinning medication.

YEAST INFECTIONS

Candida albicans is a yeast infestation that thrives in warm-blooded animals. It is scientifically classified as a fungus. This fungus can cause:

- Thrush: white patches on the inside of the mouth, inflamed red patches in the skin, bad breath, a heavily coated tongue, and a dry mouth.
- Vaginal infections: vaginal itching, pain, thick yellow discharge, and burning during urination.
- A chemical reaction in your body.
- False estrogen, which makes the body think it has enough estrogen and signals it to cease production. It also sends a message to the thyroid, making it think it has enough thyroxin and to thus stop

producing thyroxin. These results can cause menstrual irregularities and hypothyroid problems.

- An alcohol called ethanol. Ethanol can produce an intoxicated effect, if the blood count is high enough. Ethanol grows rapidly when yeast has a food source, such as white sugar or white flour products.
- In severe cases, it produces more than the liver can oxidize and eliminate.
- Acetaldehyde is another by-product of candida. It is related to formaldehyde and causes many malfunctions of the body.
- It disrupts collagen production and fatty acid oxidation, and blocks normal functions.
- It interferes with the normal function of the whole body.

As this single-cell fungus multiplies, it develops toxins that circulate in the bloodstream and causes all types of illnesses. Candida albicans is a very serious disease if allowed to thrive and left untreated. It can cause a chemical reaction in your body.

ROOT CAUSES

- Prolonged or frequent use of antibiotics or corticosteroids leading to a depletion of good bacteria.
- Poor digestion and elimination.
- A depressed immune system.
- A high-sugar diet.
- Allergies.
- Stress.
- Hormonal changes and birth control pills.
- Aging.

SYMPTOMS OF SYSTEMIC CANDIDIASIS

- Persistent fatigue, congestion, cough.
- Headaches, numbness, or tingling in the limbs.

- Diarrhea, constipation, abdominal pain.
- Colitis, rectal itching.
- Poor memory and concentration.
- Mood problems (depression, anxiety).
- Kidney and bladder infections.
- Muscle pain, allergies.
- Arthritis, chronic skin rashes.
- Canker sores, genital or toe rashes.

DIET

Base your meals around fresh vegetables, whole grains, quality sources of lean protein, and green drinks. Drink eight glasses of water daily to help flush your system.

FOODS TO AVOID

- Sugar, yeast, and all foods containing alcohol.
- Foods with mold (aged cheese, nuts, and nut butter).
- Refined foods that are likely to be loaded with sugars.
- Reduce the use of fruits and fruit juices during the initial phase.

HERBAL RECOMMENDATIONS

Eat foods such as garlic, onions, chlorella, and wheatgrass.

Pau d'arco (tabebuia avellanedae) has strong antibacterial and antifungal properties. No matter what kind of candida infection you have, drink several cups of this tea every day.

- Peppermint (mentha piperita) oil relieves intestinal cramping often associated with candida.

- Wormwood (artemisia absinthium), Oregon grape (berberis aquifolium), and rosemary (rosmarinus officinalis) all have antifungal properties.
- Tea tree oil (melaleuca alternifolia) is mainly used topically for skin-related yeast infections. The tincture form can be mixed in water (five to fifteen drops) and swished in the mouth for treating thrush.
- A high-potency multivitamin provides the many nutrients used to support detoxification.
- Vitamin C is used to enhance immune function. Take 1,000 mg two to three times daily.
- Stress reduction. High levels of stress have been implicated in candida infections. If you are prone to candida, any stress-reduction technique is likely to help.

OTHER RECOMMENDATIONS

- Change your toothbrush monthly to avoid re-infecting yourself.
- Wear cotton underwear and loose clothing to keep the area dry.

DIETARY APPROACH TO THE COMMON COLD AND FLU

Dr. David A. J. Tyrrell, a retired director of the common cold unit of the British Medical Research Council in Salisbury, England, states that "the common cold is caused by any of several hundred different viruses specially adapted to grow in the nose (rhinoviruses and coronaviruses)." Cold is spread when you inhale tiny virus-laden droplets of mucus and saliva, liberated by the sneeze or cough of an infected person. Cold can also be spread by hand-to-hand contact or infected object then touching your face with your germ-laden hands. You can avoid catching a cold by not having direct contact with an infected person and by washing your hands often.

HOW TO TREAT A COMMON COLD

There is no way to cure a cold but there are ways to make the symptoms more bearable, such as the following:

- Drink lots of fluids to keep the mucus membrane moist.
- Soothe the affected throat with warm drinks, or gargle with salt and water.
- Inhale water vapour from a humidifier, or take a hot bath or shower to help clear nasal passages. A hot bath is relaxing, as well.
- "Grandma's chicken soup." "Hot chicken soup raises the temperature in your nose and throat, creating an inhospitable environment for viruses that prefer cooler, drier climates. This hot soup also thins out mucus so you can blow it out easier. It also inhibits the growth of WBC cells (neutrophils), thus halting the development of the cold. In the Nebraska study, vegetable soup was just as effective for slowing neutrophil activity in the common cold and flu." You can add garlic to the chicken soup. Its pungent cloves contain illicit, a potent antimicrobial that can fend off bacteria. Cayenne pepper in your soup will help get the body fluid flowing, which in turn will drain stuffy sinuses.
- Ginger tea is known to boost immune-system activity and may help to beat your cold.
- According to herbalists, goldenseal and Echinacea are the dynamic cold-fighting duo. Goldenseal is a natural choice because it's loaded with berberine, a botanical antibiotic. Take one-half to one teaspoonful of goldenseal tincture twice a day, or you can take a goldenseal capsule.
- Echinacea, the popular herbal cold remedy, stimulates the immune system to fight an infection before it causes congestion and chills.
- Drugs can't cure the cold but they will make you more comfortable. Aspirin, ibuprofen, and acetaminophen will ease your body aches and pains and bring down the fever. A decongestant will make breathing easier. An expectorant cough medicine will loosen mucus in your lungs.

CHAPTER SEVEN

MEN'S HEALTH

The prostate gland is the most valuable organ of the male reproductive system. The prostate is the most common site of disorders in the male genitourinary system. The prostate gland is that part of the male reproductive system that wraps around the male urethra near the bladder. Some common problems of the prostate are:

- Benign Prostatic Hyperplasia (BPH);
- Prostate cancer.

BENIGN PROSTATIC HYPERPLASIA (BPH)

- Some of the symptoms are:
- Difficulty in starting the flow of urine.
- Weak stream of urine.
- Stopping and starting during urination and dribbling afterward.
- Among the more severe symptoms, an urgent need to urinate up to several times per hour
- A constant feeling of fullness in the bladder.
- Frequently awakening at night to go to the bathroom.

WHAT IS THE CAUSE OF BPH?

Dr. Alvin C. Powers, chief of endocrinology and diabetes at the Nashville VA Medical Center and associate professor of Medicine at Vanderbilt University, states, "There are two contributing factors for BPH: maybe insufficient consumption of grains and beans and other isoflavone-containing food, and excessive consumption of animal fat and protein." Benign prostatic hyperplasia (BPH) is very prevalent; however, prostate cancer gets lots of media coverage.

HELP FOR BENIGN PROSTATIC HYPERPLASIA:

- The goals of BPH therapy are to improve urinary flow and reduce symptoms.
- *Lifestyle changes.* If your symptoms are relatively mild, you can wait and simply monitor your condition, a "watchful wait." Be sure to check with your doctor at least once a year to make sure you are not developing complications that may harm your kidneys or bladder.
- *Saw palmetto* is very effective against urinary problems associated with an enlarged prostate, according to Dr. Leonard Ask, clinical associate professor of urology at University of Los Angeles's School of Medicine. It has been shown to shrink swollen prostate tissue and has no effect on testosterone levels; therefore, it will not diminish libido.
- *Zinc.* Zinc will help to relieve symptoms of BHP.
- *No caffeinated drinks after five p.m.* Caffeine causes you to urinate, which can be very annoying in the middle of the night.
- Limit or eliminate fluid intake between dinner and bedtime.
- *Avoid OTC antihistamines and decongestants.* These can worsen BPH by preventing muscles in the bladder and prostate from relaxing to let urine flow out.

- *Regular exercise.* For example, a study in the *Archives of Internal Medicine* reports that men who walk two to three hours a week have a 25% lower risk of developing BPH.

ERECTILE DYSFUNCTION (IMPOTENCE)

Erectile dysfunction (ED), also known as impotence, is a man's inability to maintain a firm erection long enough to have sex. This condition is common in older men but it can occur at any age. The cause is more physical than psychological. A variety of different diseases may cause ED:

- Vascular disease refers to blood vessels. These include atherosclerosis (hardening of the arteries), hypertension, and high cholesterol. These diseases are related to 70% of the physical causes of ED, since they restrict the flow of urine to the penis.
- Diabetes.
- Kidney disease.
- Neurological disease, such as multiple sclerosis or Parkinson's disease.
- Prostate enlargement.
- Prostate cancer.
- Spinal cord injury.
- Hormonal imbalances.
- Drug use.

Just a note of caution to men: according to Dr. Kenneth Goldberg, director of the Male Health Center in Lewisville, Texas, "twenty-five percent of men who see a doctor for impotence caused by vascular problems have a heart attack or stroke within five years of the start of the impotence." The reason? Sexual impotence is often caused by the same problem that causes heart trouble, including diabetes, smoking, high blood pressure, and high cholesterol levels." (Please take responsibility for your health.)

Reader's Digest Stealth Health by Dr. Debra L. Gordon and David L. Katz states, "Sex is good for you. Regular sex increases immunity from viruses, relieves stress, and even helps protect the health of a man's prostate gland by emptying fluids kept there."

CHAPTER EIGHT

WOMEN'S HEALTH

MENOPAUSE

Menopause is a normal condition that all women experience as they age. This term is used to describe the changes a woman experiences just before or after she stops menstruating, marking the end of her reproductive period. At this stage, the ovaries have stopped releasing eggs and producing most of the estrogen. Western medicine focuses on menopause as a disease that must be treated, rather than a natural change in a woman's life. Women who don't take their estrogen pills, Western medicine implies, will lose their femininity and their value to society. Luckily, many women instinctively know better and studies have proven that there are extreme health risks associated with synthetic hormone replacement. To these wise women, menopause is a time of freedom from the menstrual cycle and the onset of wisdom and power.

SYMPTOMS OF MENOPAUSE

- *Irregularly skipped period or cessation of periods.* Your period may come more or less often. It may last more or fewer days and may sometimes be lighter and sometimes heavier. Eventually, it stops.

- *Hot flashes*. As **estrogen** is involved in regulating your body temperature, without it your body acts like a house with a broken thermostat. Not enough estrogen means hot flashes. You may have sudden feelings of heat all over or in the upper part of your body. You may have flushing of the face and neck. Some women will have red blotches on their chest, back, or arms. Others have heavy sweating and cold shivering after the flash.
- *Mood swings*. Women cry more often and feel crappy.
- **Fatigue**.
- **Depression, anxiety**, and **panic attacks**.
- **Irritability**.
- **Racing heart**.
- **Headaches**.
- **Joint** and **muscle aches** and pains.
- *Changes in libido* and changing feelings about sex. Feeling less interested in sex.
- *Vaginal dryness*. Changing hormonal levels can lead to drier and thinner vaginal tissue, which makes sex uncomfortable. Some women get more infections in the vagina.
- *Bladder control*. Some women get more urinary tract infections; others have urinary incontinence.
- **Dizziness**.
- *Memory problems and difficulty concentrating*. When estrogen levels fall off in middle age, many women report having trouble concentrating and remembering details. A recent study found that dementia develops more often in women with low estrogen levels.
- Cold hands and feet.
- *Skin changes* (acne, facial hair, hair loss on scalp).
- *Insomnia*. Trouble sleeping during the night could be due to night sweats.
- *Obesity*. During menopause and as you get older, your metabolism slows down and it is easy to start packing on weight.

MANAGING MENOPAUSE SYMPTOMS

- *Be active and eat healthily.* Before menopause, women are protected against a number of diseases — such as heart disease, strokes, and osteoporosis — by the hormone estrogen. Once you stop producing estrogen, your risk of contracting these diseases increases. Being physically active and having a good diet can help protect against them. Low estrogen levels also affect other parts of the body such as your bladder, skin, and hair.
- *Increase consumption of soybeans, tofu, miso, and flaxseeds,* all of which are excellent sources of phytoestrogens. (Japanese women have significantly fewer problems during menopause because they consume foods with phytoestrogens).
- *Reduce the amount of saturated fat* (hard fat). Choose olive oil or rapeseed oil. Omega-3 is very good for your heart. Oily fish such as sardines, mackerel, herring, kippers, and salmon are good sources of fat.
- *Increase your fibre.* Soluble fibre can help lower cholesterol and reduce your risk of heart disease. This type of fibre is often found in oats, barley, pulses, and some fruits and vegetables.
- Drink plenty of water.
- *Remember vitamin E-regulated estrogen production.* Make sure to include cold-pressed nut and seed oils in your diet, perhaps as a dressing for a green salad.
- *Consume one to two tablespoons of ground flaxseeds daily.* They contain lignans, which are phytonutrients that have estrogen.
- Eat at least five portions of fruits and vegetables a day.
- Lower your salt intake.
- *Look after your bones.* As men and women age, they start to lose calcium from their bones. At menopause, women tend to lose it faster. This calcium loss results in bones getting weaker and thinner, especially at the hip and the wrist. As bones continue to thin, osteoporosis may develop. A good calcium-rich diet, along with vitamin D and plenty of weight-bearing activity, is the best thing you can do to protect yourself.

• If you smoke, quit.

WRINKLES

Your skin is your largest organ and so it's a huge target for free radicals. A lack of adequate fluid in the body causes the skin to be dry and that can contribute to the formation of wrinkles. Wrinkles form when the skin thins and loses its elasticity. As you age, your body naturally produces less collagen and elasticity (connective tissue that make your skin firm and supple). The layer of fat under your skin also begins to disappear. As a result, the skin, especially in the face, starts to sag and wrinkle. The first signs of wrinkles usually appear in the delicate tissues around the eye — smile lines or crow's feet. The cheeks and lips show damage next, but there are other factors that contribute to the formation of wrinkles, such as:

• diet and nutrition;
• muscle tone;
• habitual facial expression;
• stress;
• proper skin care;
• exposure to environmental pollutants and sun rays Exposure to the sun not only dries out the skin, it leads to free radical damage to the skin cells. The sun is the worst enemy for the skin. The ultraviolet rays that cause the actual damage are present in all seasons. These rays erode the elasticity of the skin that causes the wrinkles;
• Skin care (or lack of it);
• lifestyle habits, such as smoking;
• heredity;

SMART EATING FOR SMOOTHER SKIN

According to Dr. Mark L. Wahlqvist, an Australian researcher at Monash University in Melbourne, "certain foods can, actually, protect your face from wrinkles." He found that foods containing powerful antioxidants, whether in the form of vitamins, carotenoids, polyphenols, or other phytochemicals, can counteract dangerous free radicals.

Wahlqvist and his team of researchers learned that these foods seem to fight wrinkles: Eggs, yogurt, spinach, eggplant, asparagus, celery, garlic, onions, nuts, lima beans, olives, cherries, grapes, melons, prunes, dried fruit, apples, multigrain bread, jam, tea, and water. Olive oil contains monounsaturated fat, which resists skin cell damage, and is also very good.

AVOID WRINKLE-CAUSING FOODS

Researchers have also discovered that certain foods seem to encourage wrinkles:

Milk (full-fat), margarine, red meat, soft drinks, butter, ice cream, potatoes, cakes, pastries. Saturated fat does not protect against sun damage, and sugary products actually deteriorate your overall skin health.

RECOMMENDATIONS TO PROTECT YOUR SKIN

- Eat a well-balanced diet that includes many and varied fruits and vegetables, preferably raw; also, eat whole grains, seeds, nuts, and legumes.
- Exercise your face. Stretch the muscles under your chin and the front of your neck. Lying on a slant board for fifteen minutes a day is also good.
- Drink at least two quarts of water daily, even if you do not feel thirsty. This helps to keep the skin hydrated and flush away toxins, discouraging the formation of wrinkles.
- Get regular exercise. Like other organs of the body, skin gets its nourishment from the bloodstream. Exercise increases the circulation of the blood to the skin.

- Avoid alcohol-based toning products. Use witch hazel or an herbal/floral water instead.
- Pay attention to your facial expression. If you find yourself squinting, raising your eyebrows or making some other potentially wrinkle-inducing expression over and over again, make a conscious effort to stop it.
- Practice good skin care and keep your skin well hydrated.
- Avoid using harsh soaps or solid cleansing creams on your face. Use natural oils, such as avocado oil, to remove dirt and old make-up. Apply it gently and wash your face with warm water.
- Do not apply heavy oils around the eyes before going to bed. This may cause the eye to be puffy in the morning.
- Select good skin-care products and avoid those that contain petrolatum, mineral oil, or any hydrogenated oils. Allantoin, a soothing agent derived from comfrey, is a good ingredient to use.

CHAPTER NINE

NATURAL REMEDIES FOR SOME COMMON AILMENTS

We are living on a poisoned planet with so many man-made chemicals in our environment. Some of the foods we are consuming are genetically modified, and this food is also fed to livestock. It is no wonder we have so many health-related problems in our society today. I will briefly discuss a few of them.

ACNE

This condition is caused by overactive oil glands. Pores are blocked with metabolic toxins, and these result in whiteheads, blackheads, and inflamed pustules. This condition is caused by an improper diet, ineffective digestion, and a hormonal imbalance. With proper diet and natural remedies, you will see improvement in four to eight weeks.

- Discover and eliminate the food that will cause acne.
- A diet that's low in fat and sugar, and features plenty of water, fresh fruits, and vegetables.
- Supplements: vitamin A, vitamin C, zinc, niacin (NO flush), and vitamin E for wound healing.

- Herbal: milk thistle is excellent for detoxifying the liver and skin, Angelica/Dong Quai for hormonal balancing, Pau d'Arco helps to purify the blood.
- Skin treatment: Use cream containing vitamins A, C, and E that can penetrate the epidermis, along with Pau d'Arco cream.

ALLERGIES

Allergies are a hypersensitivity to substances that are ordinarily harmless. Genetic engineering is now increasing the levels of naturally occurring allergens already present in our food. It is very difficult to find out if our food is genetically engineered because there are requirements for labelling them.

The only thing you can do is identify the responsible allergen and avoid using it.

PESTICIDE EXPOSURE

Pesticide is a poison used to destroy pests of any sort. GMO crops are manufactured with a gene for pesticide resistance, meaning that they are sprayed with pesticides. Some of the pesticides are linked to such health problems as birth defects, cancer, diabetes, and Alzheimer's disease. The only way to protect yourself is to become very conscious of what you are putting in your mouth.

ALZHEIMER'S DISEASE

Alzheimer's disease is one of a group of brain disorders called dementia. The disease is named for Dr. Alois Alzheimer, a German doctor who, during an autopsy in 1906, discovered physical changes in the brain of a woman who had died of a strange mental illness. He found plaques and tangles in her brain, signs that are now considered the hallmark of Alzheimer's disease.

Alzheimer's disease is an irreversible, progressive brain disease that slowly destroys memory and thinking skills and eventually even the ability to carry out the simplest task.

WARNING SIGNS AND SYMPTOMS OF ALZHEIMER'S

According to the Alzheimer Society of Canada, "There is currently no cure for Alzheimer's disease and no treatment that will stop its progression. Several drugs are available that can help with some symptoms. Non-pharmacological treatment may also benefit people with Alzheimer's disease."

"Early diagnosis keeps your life from unraveling. Recognize the symptoms and why it is important to see your doctor. You can explore treatments that may provide some relief of symptoms and help you maintain a level of independence longer."

There is no definitive evidence yet about what can prevent Alzheimer's or age-related cognitive decline. However, we can reduce our risks by some of the home remedies of Alzheimer's disease.

STRESS MANAGEMENT FOR ALZHEIMER'S DISEASE

Stress that is chronic or severe takes a heavy toll on the brain, leading to shrinkage in a key memory area known as the hippocampus, hampering nerve cell growth, and increasing your risk of Alzheimer's disease and dementia. Try these proven techniques:

- *Deep breathing exercises.* Stress alters your breathing rate and impacts oxygen levels in the brain. Restorative, deep abdominal breathing is powerful, simple, and free.

- *Schedule daily relaxation activities.* Keeping stress under control requires regular effort. Make relaxation a priority, whether it is a walk in the park, yoga, or a soothing bath.
- *Nourish inner peace.* Various studies associate spirituality — regular meditation, listening to special music, religious practice, and prayer — with better brain health.

BRAIN BOOSTER

According to the Alzheimer's Research and Prevention Foundation, regular physical exercise reduces your risk of developing Alzheimer's disease by 50%. Regular exercise can also slow further deterioration in those who have already started to develop cognitive problems. Look for small ways to start any type of movement in your day. For example:

- Park you vehicle at a far end of the parking lot and walk.
- Take the stairs.
- Walk around the block.
- Carry your own groceries.
- Protect your head from injury (studies reveal that head trauma at any point in life significantly increases your risk for Alzheimer's disease).

It is also a good strategy to:

- *Learn something new.* Learn sign language, a foreign language, or a musical instrument. Read a good book or the newspaper.
- *Practice memorization.* Start with something short like a poem or Bible verses.
- *Enjoy strategy games, puzzles and riddles.* Brain teasers and strategy games provide a great mental workout, and build your capacity to form and retain cognitive associations. Do a crossword puzzle, play board games or cards, or work through words and numbers games, such as Scrabble or Sudoku.

- *Practice the 5 Ws.* Observe and report like a crime detective. Keep a "who, what, where, when, and why" list of your daily experiences. Capturing visual details keeps your neurons firing.
- *Give up smoking and drinking.* Mt. Sinai Medical Center warns that a combination of these two behaviours reduces the age of Alzheimer's onset by six to seven years. When you stop smoking, the brain benefits from improved circulation almost immediately, no matter your age. However, brain changes from alcohol abuse can only be reversed in the early stages.

According to the National Institutes of Health, "In one ground-breaking study, older adults who received as few as ten sessions of mental training not only improved their cognitive functioning in daily activities in the months after the training, but continued to show long-lasting improvement ten years later."

ANXIETY

According to the *Encyclopaedia and Dictionary of Medicine and Nursing*, anxiety is a feeling of uneasiness, apprehension, or dread. Most people will find a healthy way to deal with this anxiety by sharing what they are feeling with parents, friends, and counsellors. Anxieties may begin to interfere with daily functions like work, school, social activities, and relationships.

CAUSES

Some physical health conditions are also associated with anxiety:

- Heart disease
- Hypothyroidism or hyperthyroidism
- Menopause

RISK FACTORS

- *Being female.* More than twice as many women as men are diagnosed with generalized anxiety disorder.
- *Childhood trauma.* Children who endured abuse or trauma, including witnessing traumatic events, are at higher risk of developing generalized anxiety disorder.
- *Illness or a chronic health illness such as cancer.* This can lead to constant worry about the future, your treatment, and your finances.
- *Stress.* A big event or a number of smaller stressful life situations may trigger excessive anxiety.
- *Personality.* People with some personality types are more prone to anxiety disorder than others.
- *Genetics.* Generalized anxiety disorder may run in families.
- *Substance abuse.* Drug or alcohol abuse can worsen generalized anxiety disorder.

COMPLICATIONS

Generalized anxiety disorder can lead to other mental and physical health conditions such as:

- depression;
- substance abuse;
- trouble sleeping (insomnia);
- digestive or bowel problems;
- headaches;
- teeth grinding (bruxism).

TREATMENT

- Your family doctor may prescribe antidepressants or may refer you to a psychiatrist.

- Psychotherapy (talk therapy) and psychological counselling may be ordered. This involves working out underlying life stresses and concerns, and making behaviour changes. This can be very effective for anxiety.
- Lifestyle changes can make a difference. Here are a few things that can be done:
- Get daily exercise. Exercise is a powerful stress reducer, can improve your mood and can keep you healthy. Develop a regular routine and work out most days of the week. Start out slowly.
- Diet changes. Avoid stimulants containing caffeine such as coffee, black tea, soda pop, and chocolate.
- Limit refined sugar intake.
- Eat small, frequent meals during the day. This will help to balance the blood sugar and decrease anxiety symptoms.
- Detoxification. Consider doing a three-day juice fast (made from vegetables, as too may fruit juices can give you unwanted sugar shock). Stress in the system can result from toxins; stress itself is poisonous to your system.
- Valerian is a strong nerve relaxer, and is especially helpful for insomnia caused by anxiety. Make sleep a priority.
- Certain supplements may help relieve anxiety:
- Chamomile and oat straw are great herbal nerve relaxers.
- Vitamin B and folic acid may relieve anxiety by affecting the production of chemicals needed for your brain to function (neurotransmitters).

COPING AND SUPPORT

- Join an anxiety support group.
- Work with your mental health provider, if you have one, to figure out what is making you anxious and address it.
- Let it go. Do not dwell on past problems or concerns. Change what you can and let the rest take its course.
- Stick to your treatment plan.

- Socialize. Don't let worries isolate you from loved ones or enjoyable activities. Social interaction and caring relationships can lessen your worries.

PREVENTION

- *Get help.* Early intervention is best.
- *Keep a journal.* Keeping track of your personal life can help your mental health provider to identify what's causing you stress and what seems to make you feel better.
- *Prioritize your life.* You can reduce anxiety by carefully managing your time and energy.
- *Avoid unhealthy substance use.* Alcohol, drugs, caffeine, and nicotine can cause or worsen anxiety.

BAD BREATH (HALITOSIS)

Bad breath is the foul smell from rotten food in the digestive tract, caused by constipation. It can also be caused by a liver problem, tooth decay (inadequate dental care), inadequate protein digestion, foreign bacteria in the mouth, gum, throat, or nose, infection, indigestion, improper diet, and/or poor food combination. It can also be a sign of other health problems.

OTHER CAUSES OF BAD BREATH:

- The type of food you eat. Garlic, onion, fish, fats, and meat are big culprits. (Even when these foods are digested, the volatile chemicals that are absorbed in your bloodstream are carried to your lungs where they are exhaled in your breath.)
- Smoking.
- Alcohol.
- Dentures.

- Chronic lung or sinus infections.
- Not brushing or flossing daily.
- Systemic diseases such as diabetes and kidney disorders.
- Periodontal or gum disease.
- Taking certain medications.

TREATMENT AND PREVENTION

- Proper care of the mouth and teeth and regular visits to your dentist are important.
- Daily brushing and flossing. You should brush three times and floss daily.
- Keep your nose and sinuses clean.
- Diet. A healthful source of fibre including whole grains, raw or lightly cooked fruits and vegetables, beans, raw nuts, and seeds will improve your digestive system's ability to process food and expel toxins.
- Detoxification. To get rid of undigested foods, go on a three-day juice fast. Emphasize green drinks during your fast and go easy on juices made with sweet fruits.
- Chlorophyll. Green drinks are one of the best ways to combat bad breath. Chlorophyll cleanses the bloodstream and colon, which can be the site where bad breath begins. Chlorophyll can also be used as a mouth rinse.
- Drink at least eight glasses of water daily to keep your mouth moist and to help rinse away odour-forming bacteria.
- Cut out alcohol and coffee.
- Prevent hunger breath by eating regularly.
- Vitamin C — 2,000 to 6,000 mg daily — is vital in healing mouth and gum disease, and rids the body of excess mucous and toxins that can cause bad breath.
- Garlic capsules act as a natural antibiotic, destroying foreign bacteria in both the mouth and colon.
- Vegetarian acidophilus balances "friendly" bacteria in the colon.

- Avoid foods that take a long time to travel through the digestive system. Red meat, fried foods, and processed foods all linger in the system, and cause both constipation and halitosis. Cut down on mucus-forming foods, like dairy products, refined flours, chocolate, and bananas. Foods that are most likely to cause temporary bad breath include garlic, onions, strong cheese, cured meats, and anchovies. If the resulting odour bothers you, limit or stop your consumption of these items.

CARPAL TUNNEL SYNDROME

According to the National Institute of Neurological Disorders and Stroke, "Carpal tunnel syndrome occurs when the median nerve, which runs from the forearm into the palm of the hand, becomes pressed or squeezed at the wrist. The median nerve controls sensations to the palm side of the thumb and fingers (although not the little finger), as well as impulses to some small muscles in the hand that allow the fingers and thumb to move. The carpal tunnel — a narrow passageway of ligament and bones at the base of the hand, houses the median and tendons."

Symptoms of carpal tunnel syndrome usually start gradually with the following:

- Frequent pain in arm or hand with weakness.
- Tingling numbness in the palm of the hand and fingers.
- Difficulty clenching the fist or grasping small objects.

CAUSES OF CARPAL TUNNEL SYNDROME

- A combination of factors that increase pressure on the median nerve and tendons.
- A cyst in the carpal tunnel.
- Edema/fluid retention.

- Hypothyroidism (underactive thyroid gland).
- Diabetes.
- Obesity.
- Degenerative rheumatoid arthritis.
- Overactive pituitary gland.
- Work stress.

TREATMENT OF CARPAL TUNNEL SYNDROME

- Treatment should begin as early as possible.
- Stop, limit, or modify the activity that stimulates the discomfort.
- Pain can be relieved by shaking the hands vigorously or dangling the arms.
- Acupuncture, osteopathy, or chiropractic treatment many be helpful.

DIARRHEA

Diarrhea describes bowel movements (stools) that are loose and watery. Everyone will experience diarrhea sometime in their life. Diarrhea generally lasts for a day or two; however, it can last for weeks. In these situations, it can be a sign of a serious disorder, such as inflammatory bowel disease or irritable bowel syndrome.

SYMPTOMS OF DIARRHEA

- Frequent, loose, watery bowel movements.
- Abdominal cramps and pain.
- Nausea and vomiting.
- Fever.
- Dehydration.
- Blood in stool (sometimes).
- Bloating.

WHEN TO SEE YOUR DOCTOR

- Diarrhea lasts for more than two days.
- You become dehydrated. When you are very thirsty, your mouth is dry, you produce little or no urination or the urine is dark, you experience severe weakness, dizziness, or light-headedness.
- You have severe rectal pain.
- You have bloody or black stools.
- You have a fever above 102 F (39 C).

DIARRHEA IN CHILDREN

COMMON CAUSES OF DIARRHEA IN CHILDREN

- Infection from viruses like rotavirus or bacteria like salmonella. Viruses are the most common cause of a child's diarrhea.
- Medications like laxatives and antibiotics can also lead to diarrhea.
- Food poisoning. Symptoms of food poisoning will go away in 24 hours.

TREATMENT FOR DIARRHEA

- Prevent and replace fluid loss. If it's a baby, offer additional breast-feeding or an oral rehydration solution.
- Older children should be encouraged to drink anything they like to stay hydrated.
- Studies have shown that probiotics (yogurt) can help ease diarrhea caused by antibiotics by helping to replace the healthy gut bacteria they kill.
- Call 911 if the child is too weak to stand, is confused, or dizzy.
- Take the child to the doctor right away if the child:
  - has had diarrhea more than three days;
  - is younger than six months;

- is vomiting bloody green or yellow fluid;
- can't hold down fluid or has vomited more than two times;
- has a fever over 105 F;
- seems dehydrated;
- has bloody stool;
- is less than a month old with three or more episodes of diarrhea;
- passes more than four diarrhea stools in eight hours and isn't drinking enough;
- has a weak immune system;
- has a rash;
- has stomach pain for more than two hours;
- has not urinated in six hours if a baby, or twelve hours if a child.

EAR PROBLEMS

There are many different types of ear problems. Some examples are:

- Otitis Media. This is inflammation of the middle ear, which causes a build-up of fluid with or without an infection. If an infection is present, it is often viral. Before reaching the age of seven years, many children will have several bouts of otitis media.

CAUSE OF OTITIS MEDIA

This is usually caused by bacteria or a virus that gets into the body through the nose or mouth. Some places where a number of children spend time, such as daycare centres, help the germ to spread more easily.

Other causes are:

- Respiratory infections;
- Allergies;
- Air pollutants;

- Second-hand smoke;
- Build-up of wax in the ear.

TREATMENT FOR EAR PROBLEMS

Signs and symptoms of an ear infection can indicate a number of conditions. It's important to get an accurate diagnosis and prompt treatment, **so call the doctor if:**

- Symptoms last for more than one day.
- Ear pain is severe and there is dizziness.
- Your infant or toddler is sleepless or irritable after a cold or other upper respiratory infection.
- You observe a discharge of fluid, pus, or bloody discharge from the ear.
- The child suffers an earache and feels unwell.
- The child suffered any neck or head trauma before the ear pain started.
- Hearing is acutely impaired and gradually deteriorating.
- You suspect a foreign object in the ear.
- You use a medicine for your ear and there is no improvement, but the ears become itchy.
- An adult with pain or discharge should also see a doctor as soon as possible.

ALTERNATIVE THERAPY FOR MILD EAR INFECTION

- Diet. Drinking lots of water will help to thin mucus secretion. A diet high in whole grains, protein, fresh fruits, and vegetables will build up the immune system. So will non-dairy milk and formula.
- Garlic or garlic/mullein drops. Put two drops in the affected ears three times daily. Do not use if fluid is draining from the ear.
- Echinacea and goldenseal. Adults should take four mL and children two mL four times daily to build the immune system.

- Vitamin C. Adults should take 1,000 mg three times daily; children should take 500 mg. Vitamin C enhances immune function and reduces inflammation.

SYMPTOMS OF OTITIS MEDIA

In Babies:

- Pulling and/or scratching at the ear.
- Hearing problems.
- Fever.
- Drainage from the ear.
- Difficulty sleeping.
- Crying more than usual.
- Loss of appetite.
- Irritability and vomiting.

In Older Children and Adults:

- Earache.
- Problem hearing.
- Pressure or fullness in the ear.
- Fever.
- Drainage from the ear.
- Dizziness.
- Loss of balance.
- Nausea or vomiting.

Ear wax protects the ear and is normal. However, a build-up of wax may be a problem in some adults, and may require wax-softening ear drops. Impacted ear wax does not cause an ear discharge or pain, but it may cause hearing impairment. In this case, the ear wax may need to be syringed clean by a doctor.

PREVENTING EAR PROBLEMS

- Do not use cotton swabs or other devices to clean your ears. Repeated attempts with them may result in the ear wax becoming more deeply impacted.
- Use ear plugs to prevent water going into your ear while swimming.
- Use ear protectors if you are working in a noisy environment. Blow your nose correctly. Do not squeeze the nose when blowing, and do not sniff.
- If you suspect hearing loss in a child, it is important to get it checked. Things to look for if hearing impairment is present in a child. The child:
  - is inattentive at school.
  - does not respond to instructions.
  - seems to disobey or wants the TV on loud.

GLAUCOMA

This is a disorder of the eye in which there is increased intraocular pressure, due to the imbalance in the production and the drainage of the aqueous humor. There are two main types of glaucoma:

1. Narrow angled.
2. Open angles glaucoma, the most common type.

THREE IMPORTANT POINTS IN THE MANAGEMENT OF GLAUCOMA

- Miotics drops are used to cause the pupil to constrict, thus creating a larger angle in the anterior and facilitating easier drainage of the aqueous humour.
- If conservative measures like using miotics fail, then surgery is undertaken.

- Even after surgery, miotics must be used and the client should not be out of stock of the drug because one aim in treating glaucoma is to decrease the intraocular pressure, thus giving the client a wider field of vision. Rest is also very essential.

HEADACHES

Almost everyone gets headaches sometime in their life.

Sometimes, headaches may signal a medical emergency. Seek medical attention at once if you have a headache that is much more severe than any you've had before and accompanied by the following symptoms: double vision, confusion or disorientation, a stiff neck, projectile vomiting, paralysis, vertigo, fever, deafness in one ear, extreme fatigue, or weakness. Headaches may be triggered by several factors, such as:

- Eyestrain, which can be caused by looking at the computer for too long; also, if you are wearing glasses with incorrect lens or aren't, and you need glasses.
- Diet and lifestyle, poor diet and eating habits, smoking, alcohol, caffeine, and allergies.
- Emotional stress.
- Liver toxicity.
- Dental problems.
- Low blood sugar.
- Hormonal imbalance.
- Constipation.
- Sinusitis.
- Ear problems.
- Temporomandibular joint disorders (TMJ).
- Allergies.

Cluster headache: One-sided headache that is intense for a number of days or weeks, then disappears and reappears later.

Tension headache: Sensation of a tight band around the head, pressure or throbbing anywhere in the head or neck and tension in the neck or shoulder.

Migraine headache: Severe pain, usually on one side of the head, with vision disturbances that proceed or accompany the headache. Sensitivity to light, nausea, and vomiting. This may last for several days.

TREATMENT

First, you have to find the cause of the headache and try to evaluate it. A toxic system is one of the many causes of headaches. Relieving the system of toxic waste can alleviate headaches and leave you feeling refreshed and strong.

A gentle herbal cleanse can work magic for headaches.

Other recommendations include the following:

- Eat a diet rich in whole foods, which means eating foods that are close as possible to how nature made them. Eat your fruits raw, not canned or frozen. Eat your vegetables raw or lightly steamed or sautéed. Use organically grown eggs, meats, and fresh fish in your diet. Make sure you eat a piece of raw fruit and a vegetable at every meal.
- Get enough fibre to keep the bowels regular and reduce toxic build-up.
- Drink a glass of clean water every two waking hours, to keep the muscles in the head and neck supple, and to flush out toxins from the body.

- Include sources of magnesium and calcium in your diet. Calcium relaxes the nervous system, the muscles, and blood vessels, making it helpful for all types of headaches but especially tension headaches. Soy products, green, leafy vegetables, and beans are all rich in calcium. Green, leafy vegetables are good sources of magnesium, as well as nuts, bananas, and wheat germ. Fish are rich in omega-3 fatty acids that can help to prevent migraines.
- Take a few quiet moments with a relaxing cup of tea such as peppermint, chamomile, and passionflower.
- Melatonin has been shown in preliminary research to help migraine headaches. This is a hormonal supplement that also helps insomnia.
- Deep breathing exercises. Some headaches are caused by an inadequate supply of oxygen.
- A heating pad, a warm compress, or a hot towel on the back of the neck or the shoulders is a relaxing way to relieve tension.

FIBROIDS

Uterine fibroids are noncancerous growths of the uterus that usually appear during the childbearing years. They develop from smooth muscle tissue of the uterus (myometrium). A single cell divides repeatedly, eventually creating a firm, rubbery mass distinct from nearby tissue. Fibroids range in size from seedlings to bulky masses that can distort and enlarge the uterus. They can be single or multiple. Many women with fibroids are unaware of them because they cause no symptoms. They are sometimes found during routine examinations.

SYMPTOMS OF FIBROIDS

- Enlarged abdomen.
- Fibroid tumors can press against neighbouring organs such as the intestines or bladder, causing constipation or difficulty passing urine.
- Pain and vaginal bleeding.

- Pelvic pressure.
- Infertility.

TREATMENT FOR FIBROIDS

Treatment of fibroids varies depending on the age of the client and the size of the growth. If the client is older and does not want children, a hysterectomy will be done. If the client is young and desires children, a myomectomy — a surgical incision in the abdomen — is done, and the tumour is removed.

FREE RADICALS

Recent research has shown that a lot of tissue damage found in heart disease, diabetes, cancer, and dementia is caused by free-radical damage, or an over-abundance of a group of loose or unpaired electrons in the body. If not controlled, these free radicals can increase the progress of aging and diseases.

SOURCES OF FREE RADICALS:

- Chemical toxins may come from antiseptic spray on vegetables and fruits, electric waste, and other sources in our daily life.
- Ionizing radiation from the sun. Too much exposure may result in skin cancer, wrinkles, and cataracts. Even on cloudy days, we are exposed to UV light.
- X-rays.
- Industrial pollutants (toxic metals like arsenic and mercury).
- Radiation is increasing in sources around city life. Mobile phones, TVs, computers, X-rays, microwaves, and other electronic equipment expose our bodies to a lot of free radicals.
- Air pollution is a common social problem now all over the world. Emissions from factories, automobiles, and building sites lead to serious air pollution in a lot of cities.

- Pharmaceutical medications.
- People suffering a chronic illness have more free radicals than healthy individuals.
- Fried foods and high-fat diets are notorious sources of free radicals.
- Free radicals that disrupt the integrity of cell membranes are neutralized by molecules called antioxidants. Researchers have found that vitamins E and C can decrease the level of free radicals in the blood.

GOUT

I have had many of my clients come into my office complaining of pain and burning in their big toes, often stating it is very painful to walk. On examination, the toe is often warm to the touch, a bit swollen, and painful.

This acid build-up can lead to:

- Sharp uric acid crystal deposits (called tophi) in joints, often in the big toe, that look like lumps under the skin.
- Kidney stones from uric acid crystals in the kidneys.

For many people, the first attack of gout occurs in the big toe. Often, the attack wakes a person from sleep. The toe is very sore, red, warm, and swollen.

SIGNS AND SYMPTOMS OF GOUT:

- Pain;
- Swelling;
- Redness;
- Heat stiffness in the joints;
- Fever.
- In addition to the big toe, gout can affect the:

- Insteps;
- Ankles;
- Heels;
- Knees;
- Wrists;
- Fingers;
- Elbows.

A gout attack can be brought on by stressful events, alcohol, drugs, or illness.

WHAT CAUSES GOUT?

Gout is caused by the build-up of too much uric acid in the body. Uric acid is a chemical created when the body breaks down substances called purines. Purines are found in all your tissues. They are also in many foods, such as liver, dried beans and peas, and anchovies. Normally, uric acid dissolves in the blood. It passes through the kidneys and out of the body in the urine.

But uric acid can build up in the blood when:

- The body increases the amount of uric acid it makes.
- The kidneys do not get rid of enough uric acid (kidney disease).
- You eat a diet high in saturated fats, refined carbohydrates, and alcohol.
- You're insulin resistant.
- You're dehydrated.
- You're obese.
- You suffer a joint injury.
- You're under stress.
- You have high blood pressure.
- You suffer lead toxicity.
- You have an acidic system.

- Pharmaceutical medications that increase uric acid include aspirin, diuretics, cyclosporine, levodopa, and high doses of niacin.

NATURAL THERAPY FOR GOUT

Detoxification:

Start a three-day juice fast that consists of:

- Large amounts of cherry juice and green drink (wheat-grass, chlorella, spirulina, etc.)
- Plenty of water and herbal teas.

This fast will help to eliminate uric acid and reduce inflammation. Do not fast for more than three days. Long periods without food can have a reverse effect and actually raise the level of uric acid in your body. After the fast, limit yourself to raw fruits and vegetables along with juices, herbal teas, and water for several days until the pain subsides.

FOODS TO AVOID

- Eliminate foods that are high in purines, such as the following:
- Red meat, meat broths and gravies, bouillon, consommé, sweetbreads, shellfish, anchovies, herring, mushrooms, asparagus, brewer's yeast, poultry, eggs, dried beans, peas, lentils, cooked spinach, rhubarb.
- Rich foods aggravate gout pain.
- Saturated, hydrogenated, and partially hydrogenated fats and oils, and products made with refined flour or sugar.

HAIR LOSS

The hair is nourished at the root by your diet. Hair loss can be caused by diabetes, skin disease, vitamin deficiency, thyroid disease, excessive estrogen, iron deficiency, poor circulation, weight loss, acute illness, radiation, surgery, inadequate nourishment before menopause or during pregnancy, and chemotherapy. As part of the body's renewal process, most people lose 50 to 100 hairs every day. The average rate of growth is approximately a half inch per month. Hair grows fastest in the summer. Most rapid hair loss begins in both sexes by the age of fifty. Genetics and hormones determine the most common reason for hair loss.

TREATMENT

- *Diet.* Eat varied, well-rounded meals made from basic food including plenty of whole grains, vegetables, and quality protein (beans, nuts, fish, and lean poultry).
- *Biotin* promotes hair and scalp health and, in some cases, can prevent hair loss. Some sources of biotin are nuts, brown rice, brewer's yeast, and oats. Many of these foods are high in the vitamin Bs, which promote hair growth.
- *Iron* is essential for hair growth. Include the following foods in your diet: green, leafy vegetables, leeks, cashews, berries, dried foods, and figs.
- Your body needs *vitamin C* to absorb iron and eat citrus fruits.
- Avoid foods that deplete your system of nutrients and impair circulation such as saturated and hydrogenated fats, refined flour, and sugar and processed foods.
- *Essential fatty acids,* such as omega-3, flaxseed oil and evening primrose or borage oil are beneficial. They enhance hair texture and prevent dry, brittle hair.
- Kelp-supplied minerals for hair growth.
- *Para-aminobenzoic acid* (PABA) can be used for graying hair.
- *Silica* keeps hair looking shiny and sleek.
- *Zinc* is a mineral required for hair development. Take thirty mg daily, along with three mg of copper.
- Take a *high-potency multivitamin* daily to provide the base nutrients that are required for healthy hair.

- Now that we have a better understanding of the awesome creative specimen called our bodies and realize that we cannot find a replacement for it, the only wise thing to do is to improve the care we give to ourselves.

INCONTINENCE

Urinary incontinence is the loss of bladder control. It is a common and very embarrassing condition. The severity ranges from occasional leaking when you cough or sneeze to having an urge to urinate that's so sudden and strong that you don't have sufficient time to rush to the toilet before the urine is out.

Stress incontinence occurs when you exert pressure on the bladder in stressful situations such as:

- Coughing, sneezing, laughing, exercising, or lifting something heavy. Stress incontinence occurs when the sphincter muscles of the bladder are weakened. In women, physical changes result from pregnancy, childbirth, and menopause. In men, removal of the prostate can lead to stress incontinence.
- Urge incontinence is a sudden intense urge to urinate, followed by an involuntary loss of urine. Your bladder muscle contracts and may give you a warning of only a few seconds to a minute to reach a toilet. This may be caused by:
- urinary tract infections, bladder irritants, bowel problems, Parkinson's disease, Alzheimer's disease, stroke, injury, or nervous system damage associated with multiple sclerosis.
- Overflow incontinence, when you constantly dribble urine, is the inability to fully empty your bladder. You may feel as if you never completely empty your bladder. When you urinate, you may produce only a weak stream of urine. This can affect people with damaged bladders, blocked urethras, or nerve damage from diabetes, multiple

sclerosis, or spinal cord injury. In men, this problem can be associated with prostate problems.

- Mixed incontinence is when f you experience symptoms of more than one type of urina incontinence.
- Functional incontinence happens to many older adults, especially people in nursing homes, simply because physical or mental impairment keeps them from making it to the toilet in time. For example, people with arthritis may not be able to unbutton their pants quickly enough.
- Total incontinence is the continuous leaking of urine or periodic uncontrollable leaking of large amounts of urine.

CAUSES

Urinary incontinence is not a disease, but a symptom. It can be caused by everyday habits, underlying medical conditions, or physical problems.

Some of the causes are as follows:

- *Alcohol*. Alcohol acts a bladder stimulant and a diuretic, which can cause an urgent need to urinate.
- **Over-hydration**. Drinking a lot of fluid in a short period of time increases the amount of urine your bladder has to deal with.
- **Caffeine**. This is a diuretic and a bladder stimulant that can cause the sudden need to urinate.
- **Bladder irritants**. Carbonated drinks, tea, coffee with or without caffeine, artificial sweeteners, corn syrup, and foods and beverages that are high in spice, sugar, and acid — such as citrus and tomatoes — can aggravate the bladder.
- **Medications**. Heart and blood pressure medication, sedatives, muscle relaxants, and other medications may contribute to bladder control problems.
- **Urinary tract infections**. Infection can irritate your bladder, giving you a strong urge to urinate. These urges may result in episodes of

incontinence, which may be your only warning sign of a urinary tract infection. Other possible signs and symptoms include a burning sensation when you urinate and foul-smelling urine.

- **Constipation.** The rectum is located near the bladder and shares many of the same nerves. Hard, compacted stool in your rectum causes these nerves to be overactive and increase urinary frequency. In addition, compacted stool can sometimes interfere with the emptying of the bladder, which may cause overflow incontinence.

CAUSES OF PERSISTENT URINARY INCONTINENCE

- **Pregnancy and childbirth.** Pregnant women may experience stress incontinence due to hormonal changes and increased weight pressing on the bladder.
- **Changes with aging.** After menopause, women produce less estrogen, a hormone that keeps the lining of the bladder and urethra healthy. With less estrogen, these tissues may deteriorate, which can aggravate incontinence.
- **Hysterectomy.** In women, the bladder and the uterus lie close to one another and are supported by many of the same muscles and ligaments. After surgery there may be some damage to the supporting pelvic floor, which can lead to incontinence.
- **Painful bladder syndrome** (interstitial cystitis). This chronic condition causes painful and frequent urination and rarely urinary incontinence.
- **Inflammation of the prostate gland.** Urinary incontinence sometimes occurs with this condition.
- **Enlarged prostate.** In older men, incontinence often stems from enlargement of the prostate gland.
- **Prostate cancer.** In men, stress incontinence or urge incontinence can be associated with untreated prostate cancer. Urinary incontinence is a side effect of the treatment of radiation and surgery.

- *Bladder cancer and bladder stones.* Incontinence, urinary urgency, and burning with urination can be signs and symptoms of bladder cancer or bladder stones. Others include blood in the urine and pelvic pain.
- *Neurological disorders.* Multiple sclerosis, Parkinson's disease, stroke, brain tumour, or a spinal injury can interfere with nerve signals involved in bladder control, causing urinary incontinence.
- *Obstructions.* A tumour anywhere along the urinary tract can block the normal flow of urine and cause incontinence, usually overflow incontinence. Urinary stones (hard, stone-like masses that can form in the bladder) may be to blame for urine leakage. Stones can be present in your kidneys, bladder, or ureters.

SOME RISK FACTORS

- *Sex.* Women are more likely than men to have stress incontinence.
- *Age.* As you age, the muscles in your bladder and urethra lose some of their strength.
- *Being overweight.* Being overweight increases the pressure on your bladder and surrounding muscles, which weakens them and allows urine to leak out when you cough or sneeze.
- *Smoking.* Chronic cough associated with smoking can cause episodes of incontinence.
- *Other diseases.* Kidney disease or diabetes may increase your risk for incontinence.

COMPLICATIONS

- *Skin problems.* Urinary incontinence can lead to rashes, skin infections, and sores (moisture-related skin ulcers, when urine is left on the skin too long).
- *Urinary tract infections.* Incontinence increases your risk of repeated urinary infections.

- *Changes in activities*. You may be forced to stop exercising or quit attending social gatherings.
- *Changes in your work life*. Urinary incontinence may negatively affect your work life. Your urge to urinate may cause you to get up often during meetings. This problem may disrupt your concentration at work or keep you awake at night, causing fatigue.
- *Changes in your personal life*. Your family may not understand your behaviour or may grow frustrated at your many trips to the bathroom. You may avoid sexual intimacy because of embarrassment caused by urine leakage. You may even experience anxiety and depression.

JAUNDICE

Jaundice is not a disease but a sign that can occur in many different diseases. It is a yellowish staining of the skin and sclera (the white of the eyes) that is caused by high levels of the chemical bilirubin in the blood. The colour of the skin and eyes varies depending on the level of bilirubin in the blood.

CAUSES OF JAUNDICE

Jaundice comes from the French word *jaune*, which means *yellow*. Jaundice is the yellow colour seen in the skin of many newborns. It happens when a chemical called bilirubin builds up in the baby's blood. (For the first few days after birth, the baby's liver does not work as well as it does later, so there tends to be a build-up of bilirubin in the blood). In the human body, new blood is being made all the time and old blood is being destroyed. One of the products of destroyed blood is called bilirubin. Bilirubin normally goes to the liver to be processed and then leaves the body in the feces.

Some causes of jaundice are as follows:

- **Viral hepatitis**: Hepatitis A, B, C, D, and E can all cause temporary liver inflammation. Types B and C can cause chronic life-long inflammation.
- **Autoimmune hepatitis**: In this condition, the body's immune system attacks its own liver cells. Autoimmune hepatitis is more common in people with families with other autoimmune disease such as lupus, thyroid disease, diabetes, or ulcerative colitis.
- **Alcoholic liver disease**: This involves damage to the liver caused by excessive, long-term consumption of alcohol.
- **Tumours**: These may be in the liver, pancreas, or gallbladder. They are occasionally responsible for obstruction.

SYMPTOMS OF JAUNDICE

- Yellow tinge to the skin, usually appearing first on the face and scalp.
- Yellow tinge to the white parts of the eyes (sclera).
- The urine is very dark. The body is trying to get rid of excessive bilirubin in the urine. This sign indicates poor liver function or increased red blood cell destruction.
- In babies, poor feeding and sleepiness.
- If a fever or flu-like illness comes before jaundice, it's usually a sign of a viral hepatitis infection.
- Pale, white, or clay-coloured stool indicates an obstruction in the gallbladder or bile ducts.
- Abdominal pain is felt because of the obstruction of gallstones.

NATURAL REMEDIES TO HELP WITH JAUNDICE:

There are usually very serious ailments behind adult jaundice, so you should see your doctor first to find out the cause before you start to treat yourself. In her article, "Treating Adult Jaundice Naturally," Abby Willow gives the following recommendations:

- Wheat grass is an excellent way to boost the liver with enzymatic-increasing abilities to help flush the excessive bilirubin from the body, taken once daily.
- Lime or lemon juice — ten to twenty drops in a glass of water — helps to detoxify the body.
- Dandelion tea is a natural detoxifier and diuretic, helping the body flush out excessive toxins.
- Tomato juice with a pinch of salt and pepper first thing in the morning is helpful in preventing and treating jaundice.
- Ginger is a natural detoxifier. A teaspoonful along with a teaspoonful of lime and mint will help treat jaundice with a major detoxifier boost.
- Avoiding fatty, salty, oily foods will help the body flush out toxins naturally. Keep the diet rich in calcium and iron.
- Drink herbal tea daily. Lemon, ginger, and dandelion tea helps the body flush out toxins.
- Drink at least eight glasses of water daily.

KELOID SCAR

Keloids can form after skin injuries from:

- acne;
- burns;
- chickenpox;
- ear piercing;
- cuts from surgery or trauma;
- vaccination sites.

The problem is more common in people ages ten to twenty, and in African descendants, Asians, and Hispanics. Keloids often run in families.

A keloid may be:

- flesh-coloured, red or pink;
- located over the site of a wound or injury;
- lumpy (nodular) or ridged;
- tender and itchy;
- irritated from friction such as rubbing on clothing.

TREATMENT

Keloids often do not need treatment. If the keloid bothers you, the following things can be done to reduce the size:

- Corticosteroid injections.
- Freezing (cryotherapy).
- Laser treatments.
- Radiations.
- Surgical removal.
- Silicone gel or patches.

Many of these treatments, however, can cause a larger scar to form.

PROGNOSIS

Keloids usually are not harmful to your health, but may affect how you look. In some cases, they may become smaller, flatter, and less noticeable over time.

PREVENTION

When in the sun, cover keloids and add sun block. Continue these steps for at least six months after injury for an adult, and up to eighteen months for a child.

- Imiquimod cream can be used to prevent keloids from forming after surgery, or from returning after they are removed.

LICE

Head lice are very tiny insects that can survive on the scalp. They lay eggs on the scalp and can be spread very easily.

HOW DO THEY SPREAD?

Head lice can spread very easily, especially where people are in close contact. They are common among school-aged children. They spread through direct hair-to-hair contact or indirectly by sharing things like hairbrushes, hats, combs, and headphones. They don't fly or hop, but they crawl very quickly. The lice that live on people cannot live on pets.

SIGNS AND SYMPTOMS OF HEAD LICE

- Itchy scalp;
- Nits lay very small white eggs along the hair shaft close to the scalp that look like dandruff but will not shake loose with combing.
- Visual sighting of the live bugs, living close to the scalp, often more concentrated in the warmer areas around the ears and the nape of the neck.
- Irritated red bumps or rash on the nape of the neck or around the ears.

HOW TO CHECK FOR HEAD LICE

- You need good lighting.
- They are usually found very close to the scalp, at the bottom of the neck and behind the ears.
- To look for nits, part the hair in small sections, moving from one side of the head to the other. Check carefully, looking close to the scalp.

TREATMENT

Once lice have been detected, the only way to get rid of them is to remove them. Special lice shampoo can be used to kill off live lice, but the eggs and empty casings need to be removed manually using a close-toothed nit comb.

Most over-the-counter lice treatment requires a follow-up treatment after seven days. The best, most effective method for lice removal is carefully combing through and removing each louse and nit, one by one. Leaving even one behind will quickly result in a resurgence of the population and the need to start the whole process over again.

PINK EYE

SIGNS AND SYMPTOMS OF PINK EYE

- Redness or swelling of the white of the eye or inside the eyelids.
- Increased amount of tears.
- White, yellow, or green eye discharge.
- Itchy eyes.
- Burning eyes.
- Increased sensitivity to light.
- Gritty feeling in the eye.
- Crusting of the eyelids or lashes.

CAUSES OF PINK EYE

- Virus;
- Bacteria;
- Allergens (like pet dander or dust mites);
- Irritants (like smog or swimming pool chemicals) that infect or irritate the eyelid lining.

TREATMENT

Pink eye is usually mild and will often get better on its own. It can be treated by washing the eyes with warm water and drying them with disposable tissues (to prevent the spread of infection). Severe cases need to be treated by your family doctor, and may require antibiotics or other therapy.

PSORIASIS

Psoriasis is a condition that occurs when the skin grows too rapidly. The new skin moves quickly to the surface. This is caused by faulty signals from the immune system. This is not a contagious disorder, but it can be inherited.

SIGNS AND SYMPTOMS OF PSORIASIS

- Red patches of skin covered with silvery scales.
- Small scaling spots (commonly seen in children).
- Dry, cracked skin that bleeds.
- Itching, burning, or soreness.
- Thickened, pitted, or ridged nails.
- Swollen and stiff joints
- Psoriasis patches can range from a few spots of dandruff-like scaling to major eruptions that cover large areas.
- Most types of psoriasis go through cycles, flaring for a few weeks or months, and then subsiding for a time or even going into complete remission.

CAUSES

- The cause is generally unknown, but it is thought to be related to immune system problems with cells in the body.

- The T-cell (lymphocyte) attacks healthy cells by mistake. Normally, T-cells detect and fight off foreign substances, such as viruses or bacteria.

PSORIASIS TRIGGERS

- Infections such as strep throat or skin infections.
- Injury to the skin such as cuts, scrapes, bug bites, or severe sunburn.
- Stress.
- Cold weather.
- Smoking.
- Heavy alcohol consumption.
- Certain medications such as lithium, blood pressure medications, anti-malaria drugs, and iodides.

RISK FACTORS

- Family history;
- Viral and bacterial infections;
- Stress;
- Obesity;
- Smoking.

COMPLICATIONS

- Psoriatic arthritis;
- Eye problems such as conjunctivitis, blepharitis, and uveitis;
- Obesity;
- Type 2 diabetes;
- High blood pressure;
- Cardiovascular disease;
- Metabolic syndrome;
- Parkinson's disease;
- Kidney disease;

- Low self-esteem;
- Depression;
- Social isolation.

TREATMENT

If you see your family doctor, he may prescribe one of the following treatments for you:

- Topical corticosteroids;
- Vitamin D analogues (Dovonex);
- Coal tar;
- Light therapy (natural or artificial light);
- Sunlight UVB phototherapy;
- Systemic medications;
- Oral or injected medications;

QUINSY (PERITONSILLAR ABSCESS)

This is a complication of tonsillitis. When a bacterial infection from tonsillitis spreads to the areas in the throat, then pus forms next to one of the tonsils.

SYMPTOMS OF QUINSY:

- A worsening sore throat, usually on one side.
- A high temperature of 38 C.
- Difficulty opening your mouth.
- Pain when swallowing.
- Difficulty swallowing which can lead to drooling saliva.
- Change to your voice or difficulty speaking.
- Bad breath.
- Earache on the affected side.

- Headache and feeling generally unwell.
- Swelling around your face and neck.

TREATMENT OF QUINSY

- Consult your family doctor, who may give you antibiotic.
- Proper hydration is very important.
- Rest will help to increase recovery.
- Probiotics (in addition to antibiotics) in liquid form, twice daily with meals; continue for a few days after the antibiotic therapy is completed.

RADIATION

Radiation is the transference of energy in the form of waves that travel through space or materials. Many scientists agree that radiation is dangerous at high levels. The exposure to wireless products is considered "chronic" exposure, because you are bombarded constantly at a low level rather than getting short bursts of high power. Evidence has shown that this type of exposure can be more damaging in the long run. When the body is first exposed to radiation, it reacts by strengthening the immune system. But, over long-term exposure, the immune system is gradually weakened.

Most people are affected by electromagnetic radiation. During biofeedback assessments, almost everyone shows an elevation of electromagnetic stress. In our modern technological society, we are killing ourselves from so many different areas:

- the sugar assault;
- the cancer treatment assault;
- he electromagnetic assault.

There are many forms of radiation, but for this book we will briefly discuss the following:

- cell phone;
- microwaves;
- wireless computers.

Cell phones. Some scientists believe that cell phones may increase your risk of cancer. When you use your phone, you're putting the antenna that generates the radio frequency right next to your head. A study published in the February 2011 *Journal of the American Medical Association* said such positioning could alter the brain activity. This study used a flip phone; smartphones emit even more radiation. Is this dangerous? No one knows because cell phones have only been in widespread use since the 1990s — not long enough to see long-term effects. Still, researchers advise you to play it safe: since most radiation is generated while the call is connecting, don't put it to your ear until the connection is made. Use the speaker feature when possible, and wear a wireless earpiece if you can't use a speaker.

Microwaves. The danger from microwave radiation comes if the door does not completely seal. Microwaves will heat your body just like they warm that cup of coffee. So standing near a microwave with a faulty door seal can be dangerous. Repeated slamming or simple deterioration due to age can damage the door's seal. You cannot see or smell radiation leakage, so the Food and Drug Administration advises you to be cautious. Don't stand in front of or lean on the oven while it is in use.

WIRELESS COMPUTERS

Wireless computers use very dangerous electromagnetic radiation to send signals to other computers. Studies have shown that if you can pick up your neighbour's wireless signals on your computer, that means that maybe electromagnetic radiation may be coming into your home. These radiations can cause many health problems.

HEALTH PROBLEMS CAUSED BY RADIATION

- Sleep disturbances;
- Heart palpitations;
- Tumours;
- Migraines;
- Memory loss;
- Fatigue;
- Diminished organ function;
- Hair loss.

PROTECTION AGAINST RADIATION

- Turn off the computer and other electric devices (such as printer, scanner, television, microwave) when not in use.
- Unplugging the devices is even better, because many devices still emit radiation when turned off.
- Replace wireless computers with hardwired connections.
- Cut down on the amount of electrical devices you use.
- Foods that Protect against Radiation
  - Apples and other food rich in pectin;
  - Avocados;
  - Black/green tea;
  - Broccoli;
  - Beets;
  - Coconut;
  - Ginger;
  - Chlorella;
  - Kale and other leafy greens.

Many studies have shown that the body can be protected from radiation by adopting a plant-based diet rich in colourful whole foods.

CHAPTER TEN

SEXUALLY TRANSMITTED DISEASES
and other diseases

2 Timothy 2:21: "If you keep yourself pure, you will be a special utensil for honourable use. Your life will be clean, and you will be ready for the Master to use you for every good work." Our sex life is only moral when conducted *by Biblical standards and principles.* Any type of sexual act done outside holiness perverts God's standard for morality and purity. The Bible is very clear about the consequences of sexual immorality.

Galatians 6:7-8 states, "Be not deceived; God is not mocked: for whatever a man soweth, that shall he also reap. For he that soweth to his flesh shall of the flesh reap corruption; but he that soweth to the spirit shall of the spirit reap life everlasting." This is an everlasting perpetual law created by the Almighty that affects all mankind. Cause and effect. If you treat your body the way it was *not* meant to be treated, you will suffer the consequences. Keep yourself pure:

- No sex before marriage.
- No sleeping around.
- View your body as the temple of the Lord.

You will avoid the following sexually transmitted diseases, which are infections that are transmitted from having sex with an infected person. The causes of STDs are bacteria, parasites, and viruses. There are more than 20 types of STDs including:

- Chlamydia
- Gonorrhea
- Genital herpes
- HIV/AIDS
- HPV
- Syphilis
- Trichomoniasis

Most STDs affect both men and women, but in many cases the health problem they cause can be more severe for the women. If a pregnant woman has an STD, it can cause serious health problems for the baby.

CHLAMYDIA

Chlamydia is a bacterial infection of the genital tract. There are no signs and symptoms in the early stages. Symptoms usually show up one to three weeks after exposure, and they include:

- Painful urination.
- Lower abdominal pain.
- Vaginal discharge in women.
- Discharge from the penis in men.
- Pain during sexual intercourse in women.
- Testicular pain in men.

GONORRHEA

Gonorrhea is a bacterial infection and the symptoms appear within two to ten days of exposure. Signs and symptoms of gonorrhea include the following:

- Thick, cloudy, or bloody discharge from the penis or vagina.
- Pain or burning sensation when urinating.
- Abnormal menstrual bleeding.
- Painful, swollen testicles.
- Painful bowel movements.
- Anal itching.

TRICHOMONIASIS

Trichomoniasis is a common STD caused by a microscopic, one-celled parasite called trichomonas vaginalis. The organism usually affects the urinary tract in women, but often causes no symptoms in men. Trichomoniasis typically infects the vagina in women. Signs and symptoms may include the following:

- Clear, white, greenish, or yellowish vaginal discharge.
- Discharge from the penis.
- Strong vaginal odour.
- Vaginal itching or irritation.
- Itching or irritation inside the penis.
- Pain during sexual intercourse.
- Painful urination.

HIV

HIV is an infection with the human immunodeficiency virus. HIV interferes with your body's ability to effectively fight off viruses, bacteria and fungi that cause disease. And it leads to AIDS, which is a chronic, life-threatening disease. When first infected with HIV, you may have no symptoms at all. Some people develop a flu-like illness two to six weeks after being infected. Early signs and symptoms of HIV include the following:

- Fever
- Headache
- Sore throat
- Swollen lymph glands
- Rash
- Fatigue

These early signs and symptoms usually disappear within a week to a month, and are often mistaken for another viral infection. During this period, you are very infectious. More persistent or severe symptoms of HIV infection may not appear for ten years or more after the initial infection. As the virus continues to multiply and destroy immune cells, you may develop mild infections or chronic signs and symptoms such as:

- Swollen lymph nodes (often one of the first signs of HIV infection)
- Diarrhea
- Weight loss
- Fever
- Coughing and shortness of breath

LATER-STAGE HIV INFECTION:
SIGNS AND SYMPTOMS

- Persistent, unexplained fatigue.
- Soaking night sweats.
- Shaking chills or fever higher than 100.4 F (38 C) for several weeks.
- Swelling of lymph nodes for more than three months.
- Chronic diarrhea.

- Persistent headaches.
- Unusual, opportunistic infections ("opportunistic" because they take advantage of your weakened immune system, and can cause devastating illnesses).

GENITAL HERPES

This is a highly contagious disease that is caused by a type of the herpes simplex virus (HSV). This virus enters the body through small breaks in your skin or mucous membrane. Most people with genital herpes never know they have it because the symptoms are so mild they can go unnoticed. When signs and symptoms appear, the first episode is generally the worst.

SIGNS AND SYMPTOMS:

- Small red bumps, blisters (vesicles), or open sores in the genitals, anus, and nearby areas. Pain and itching around the genital area, buttocks, and inner thighs.
- After several days, the blisters may rupture and become ulcers that ooze or bleed. Eventually, scabs form and the ulcers heal.
- In women, sores can erupt in the vaginal or external genitals, buttocks, anus, or cervix.
- In men, sores can appear on the penis, scrotum, buttocks, anus, thighs or inside the urethra, the tube from the bladder to the penis.
- Painful urination.
- Flu-like symptoms such as headaches, muscle aches, and fever, as well as swollen lymph nodes in your groin.

GENITAL WARTS (HPV INFECTION & SYMPTOMS)

Genital warts caused by the human papillomavirus (HPV) are one of the most common types of STDs.

SIGNS AND SYMPTOMS:

- Small, flesh-coloured or gray swellings in your genital area.
- Several warts close together that take on a cauliflower shape.
- Itching or discomfort in your genital area.
- Bleeding with intercourse.
- Sometimes, genital warts have no symptoms. Sometimes they are as small as one millimeter in diameter or may multiply into large clusters.
- In women, genital warts can grow on the vulva, the wall of the vagina, the area between the external genitals, and the anus.
- In men, they may occur on the tip or shaft of the penis, the scrotum, or the anus.
- Genital warts can also develop in the mouth or throat of a person who had oral sex with an infected person.

HEPATITIS

Hepatitis is a serious virus that affects your liver. The most common forms of the virus are hepatitis A, B, and C.

SIGNS AND SYMPTOMS OF HEPATITIS:

Hepatitis A, B, and C are all contagious viral infections that affect your liver. Hepatitis B and C are the most serious of the three, but each causes your liver to become inflamed. Some people never develop signs and symptoms. But for those who do, they occur after several weeks and may include:

- Fatigue;
- Nausea and vomiting;
- Abdominal pain or discomfort, especially in the area of your liver;
- Loss of appetite;
- Dark urine;
- Muscle or joint pain;
- Itching;
- Yellowing of the whites of your eyes (jaundice).

SYPHILIS

Syphilis is a bacterial infection. The disease affects your genitals, skin, and mucus membranes, but also involves other parts of your body, including your brain and heart. There are four stages of syphilis:

Primary: Signs may occur from ten days to three months after exposure.

A small painful sore (chancre) on the part of your body where the infection was transmitted — usually your genitals, rectum, tongue, or lips. A small chancre is typical, but there may be multiple sores. Signs and symptoms of primary syphilis typically disappear without treatment, but the underlying disease remains and may reappear in the second (secondary) or third (tertiary) stage.

Secondary: Signs and symptoms of secondary syphilis may begin two to ten weeks after the chancre appears and may include the following:

Rash marked by red or reddish-brown, penny-sized sores over any area of the body, including your palms and soles.

- Fever.
- Fatigue and vague feeling of discomfort.
- Soreness and aching.

These signs and symptoms may disappear within a few weeks or repeatedly come and go for as long as a year.

Latent: In some people, a period called latent syphilis — in which no symptoms are present — may follow the secondary stage. Signs and symptoms may never return, or the disease may progress into the tertiary stage.

Tertiary: Without treatment, syphilis bacteria may spread, leading to serious internal damage and death years after the original infection. Some of the signs and symptoms of the tertiary stage include:

Neurological problems. These may include stroke, infection, and inflammation of the membranes and fluid surrounding the brain and spinal cord (meningitis). Other problems may include poor muscle coordination, numbness, paralysis, deafness, and visual problems. Personality changes and dementia are also possible.

Cardiovascular problems. These may include bulging (aneurysm) and inflammation of the aorta — your body's major artery — and of other blood vessels. Syphilis may also cause valvular heart disease, such as aortic valve problems.

TREATMENT

If you suspect that you have any form of sexually transmitted disease, please see your doctor for testing. Timely diagnosis and treatment are important to avoid more delays, complications, and even death.

TONSILLITIS

Tonsillitis is an inflammation of the tonsils, which are two oval-shaped clumps of lymphoid tissue at the back of the throat. Dr. H. Winter Griffith, author of *The Complete Guide to Pediatric Symptoms, Illness and Medication*, states that the "tonsils are small at birth, enlarged during childhood, and become smaller at puberty. When not infected, tonsils help prevent infection in the sinuses, mouth and throat from spreading to other body parts. Tonsillitis is contagious."

SIGNS AND SYMPTOMS OF TONSILLITIS

- Throat pain, either mild or severe.
- Swallowing difficulty.
- Chills and fever as high as 104 F (40 C) or more.
- Swollen lymph glands on either side of the jaw.
- Headache.
- Ear pain.
- Cough (sometimes).
- Vomiting (sometimes).

CAUSES OF TONSILLITIS

- Viral or bacterial infection of the tonsils.
- Risk factors.
- Crowded or unsanitary living conditions.
- Exposure to others in public places.

TREATMENT

- Use a cool mist humidifier to relieve throat irritation and cough.
- Soothing herbal tea.
- Painkillers.
- Bed rest for two to three days.

- Increased fluid intake, while the throat is still very sore.

CALL THE DOCTOR IF:

- The symptoms worsen.
- Temperature is normal for one to two days, then rises above 101 F.
- New symptoms begin, such as nausea, vomiting, skin rash, thick nasal drainage, chest pain, or shortness of breath.
- If the child has convulsions.
- Joints become painful.
- Cough produces a discoloured sputum (green, brown, or bloody).
- If there is abscess in the throat (quinsy).

TRIGGER FINGER

Trigger finger is also known as stenosing tenosynovitis. In this condition, a finger or thumb becomes locked after it has been bent. It is difficult to straighten out without pulling on it by the other hand.

SYMPTOMS OF TRIGGER FINGER

- You may hear a click when trying to straighten the affected finger.
- There is pain and/or swelling at the base of the affected finger.
- One or more fingers may be affected. Trigger finger most commonly affects your little finger, ring finger, or thumb. It is actually most common in the right hand.

CAUSE OF TRIGGER FINGER

- The cause is often unclear; it is thought to be due to some inflammation, which causes swelling of a tendon or tendon sheath.
- A tendon is a strong tissue that attaches a muscle to a bone. In this case, the tendon comes from muscles in the forearm. It passes

through the palm and attaches to the finger bone. The muscles pulling on this tendon bend the finger toward the palm.

- A tendon sheath is like a tunnel that covers and protects parts of a tendon. Normally, the tendon slides easily in and out of the sheath as you bend and straighten the finger. In trigger finger, the tendon can slide out of the sheath when you bend your finger. However, it cannot easily slide back due to swelling. The finger remains bent unless you pull it straight with your other hand.
- Most cases occur for no apparent reason in healthy people.

TREATMENT OF TRIGGER FINGER

- Simply resting the hand and allowing any inflammation to settle may resolve the problem without the need for treatment.
- Anti-inflammatory medication.
- Splinting (placing the finger or thumb in a splint so that it remains straight may improve symptoms). Some people wear the splint at night.
- Steroid injection into the tendon sheath helps the pain. Steroids work by reducing inflammation.
- Surgery (a small cut is usually made at the base of the finger and the tendon sheath is widened). This operation is usually very successful.

COMPLICATIONS

- The risk of this surgery may be damage to the tiny nerves of the finger, causing numbness.
- Infection. There may be a small risk of the incision becoming infected.

UMBILICAL HERNIA

Umbilical hernias are most common in infants, but they can affect adults. In infants, it is very evident when they cry.

SIGNS AND SYMPTOMS OF UMBILICAL HERNIA

- A soft swelling or bulge near the navel (umbilicus), ranging from half an inch to about two inches in diameter.
- In babies, this swelling is most noticeable when the infant cries, coughs, or strains. The bulge disappears when the child is on his back or is calm.
- In children, the hernia is usually painless. In adults, the hernia may cause abdominal discomfort.

WHEN TO SEE THE DOCTOR

- If the baby appears to be in pain.
- If the baby begins to vomit.
- If the bulge becomes tender, swollen, or discoloured.

CAUSE OF UMBILICAL HERNIA

- In adults, too much abdominal pressure can cause an umbilical hernia.
- Other possible causes in adults include:
- Obesity;
- Heavy lifting;
- A long history of coughing;
- Multiple pregnancies;
- Fluid in the abdominal cavity (ascites).

RISK FACTORS

- Most common in infants, especially premature babies.
- Black babies have a higher incidence of getting umbilical hernia.
- There is a higher incidence in overweight adults and in women who have had multiple pregnancies.

COMPLICATIONS

- Complications from umbilical hernias rarely occur in children. Complications can occur when the protruding abdominal tissue becomes trapped (incarcerated) and can no longer be pushed back into the abdominal cavity. This reduces the blood supply to the section of trapped intestine, and can lead to umbilical pain and tissue damage. If the trapped portion of intestine is completely cut off from the blood supply (strangulated hernia), tissue death (gangrene) may occur. Infection may spread throughout the abdominal cavity causing a life-threatening situation.
- Adults with umbilical hernias are somewhat more likely to experience incarceration or obstruction of the intestine.
- Treatment
- Emergency surgery is the treatment of choice for such obstruction.
- Most umbilical hernias close before the age of one year.
- The doctor may push back the bulge into the abdomen. Don't try this on your own.
- Surgery will be recommended for children whose hernias:
  - get bigger after age one or two.
  - don't disappear by age four.
  - become trapped or block the intestines.

VARICOSE VEINS

Varicose veins are twisted, enlarged veins near the surface of the skin. They are commonly in the legs and ankles. They usually aren't serious, but they can sometimes lead to other problems.

CAUSE OF VARICOSE VEINS

- Old age.
- Being born with defective valves.

- Being female (hormonal changes from puberty, pregnancy, and menopause can lead to varicose veins).
- Obesity.
- Pregnancy.
- A history of blood clots in your legs.
- Standing or sitting for too long periods.
- A family history of varicose veins.

SYMPTOMS OF VARICOSE VEINS

- Aching pain that may get worse after sitting or standing for a long time.
- Throbbing or cramping in the legs.
- Heaviness in the legs.
- Swelling in the legs.
- A rash that's itchy or irritated.
- Darkening of the skin (in severe cases).
- Restless legs.

COMPLICATIONS OF VARICOSE VEINS

- **Ulcers**: Extremely painful ulcers may form on the skin near varicose veins, particularly near the ankles. Ulcers are caused by long-term fluid build-up in the tissues, caused by increased pressure of blood within affected veins. A discoloured spot on the skin usually begins before an ulcer forms. See your doctor immediately if you suspect you've developed an ulcer.
- **Blood clots**: Occasionally, veins deep within the legs become enlarged. In such cases, the affected leg may swell considerably. Any sudden leg swelling warrants urgent medical attention because it may indicate a blood clot, a common condition known medically as *thrombophlebitis*.

TREATMENT OF VARICOSE VEINS

- You should avoid standing for long periods because standing increases the pressure in the veins. Elevate the leg whenever possible, which will help circulate the blood back to the heart. Do not cross your legs when sitting.
- If you are overweight, try to lose some pounds. Obesity will increase the pressure in the legs, thereby blocking the flow of blood to the veins.
- Support from elastic stockings can provide relief from aching. This type of support helps the blood to flow back to the heart. This stocking should be put on first thing in the morning and removed before going to sleep at night.
- Walking is a very good type of exercise for varicose veins. It improves the strength in the legs and the veins.

RECOMMENDATIONS TO HELP WITH VARICOSE VEINS

- Vitamin E will prevent blood clots, a possible side effect of varicose veins.
- Red or blue coloured berries are an ideal dessert or snack for you. They fortify vein walls and improve their elasticity.
- Bilberry improves circulation and strengthens capillary walls.
- Flaxseed oil improves regularity and reduces straining. It also contains essential fatty acids that promote tissue healing.
- Witch hazel. Apply it as a gel or a cream to external varicose veins.
- Exercise to improve circulation. Ride a bike or swim.
- Wear supportive stockings.

WARTS

A wart is a skin growth caused by some types of the virus called the human papillomavirus (HPV). HPV infects the top layer of the skin, usually entering the body in an area of broken skin. The virus causes the top layer of the skin to grow rapidly, forming a wart. Most warts go away on their own within months or years.

TYPES OF WART

- Common warts: grow mainly on the hand, but can grow anywhere (raised wart with roughened surface).
- Plantar warts: a hard sometimes painful lump, often with multiple black specks in the centre; usually found on pressure points on the soles of the feet.
- Flat wart: a small, smooth, flattened wart that's flesh coloured and can occur in large numbers. It is most common on the face, neck, hands, wrist, and knees.
- Filiform or digitate wart: a thread- or finger-like wart, most common on the face, especially near the eyelids and lips.
- Genital wart: a wart that occurs on the genitalia.
- Periungual wart: a cauliflower-like cluster of warts that occurs around the nails.

WHAT CAUSES WARTS:

- Human papillomavirus (HPV). There are more than 100 types of HPV, and they cause different types of warts.
- Most types of warts, such as the common wart are harmless; others can cause serious diseases such as cancer of the cervix.
- Warts are contagious and can pass from person to person.
- Warts can be spread by coming in contact with infected towels or objects. Each person responds to the HPV virus differently; not everyone develops warts. If you have warts, you can spread the virus to other places on your own body. Warts are usually spread by broken skin such as hangnails or scrapes. Biting your nails can cause warts to spread on your fingertips and around the nails.

RISK FACTORS

- Children and young adults.
- People with weakened immune systems, such as those with HIV/AIDS or people who have had an organ transplant.

COMPLICATIONS

Because warts shed HPV, new warts can appear as quickly as old ones go away. They can also spread to other people.

TREATMENT

Common warts don't require treatment; they usually disappear within two years, although new ones may develop nearby. You may want to treat them for cosmetic purposes.

If you have stubborn warts and home treatment is not effective, your doctor may try:

- Freezing
- Minor surgery

HOME REMEDIES FOR WARTS

If mainstream methods to treat warts have not worked, try the following straightforward home remedies:

- **Apple cider vinegar**: Soak a cotton ball in apple cider and tape it over the wart. Do this every night; you will see results within one to two weeks.
- **Vitamin C**: Crush one vitamin C tablet, add lemon juice or water to make a paste. Apply paste to wart with a bandage daily until wart disappears.

- **Pineapple juice**: This juice has a high level of acidity and special enzymes to dissolve and eat away at the wart. Soak the wart in pineapple juice for three to five minutes. Dry the area after. This can be done two to three times daily until the wart is gone.

XEROPHTHALMIA

Xerophthalmia is a medical condition in which the eye fails to produce tears. It may be caused by a deficiency in vitamin A, although there may be other causes. This condition is also called dry eye syndrome. In this condition the eyes become abnormally dry because they can't maintain an adequate layer of tears to coat ther surface.

Tears are made up of:

- Water, which helps to clean the eyes and wash away dust and other foreign particles.
- Oil, which helps keep tears from evaporating too quickly.
- Mucus, which helps spread tears evenly over the surface of the eye (cornea).

If the eye does not produce enough tears or produces tears with abnormal levels of oil, water, or mucus, it can feel dry and itchy.

CAUSES OF XEROPHTHALMIA

- Wind;
- Dry air;
- Working long hours at the computer;
- Vitamin A deficiency (endemic in Third-World countries);
- Certain medication (birth control pills, antihistamines);
- Diseases such as diabetes, arthritis and Sjogren's syndrome;

- Systemic lupus erythematosus, rheumatoid arthritis, and scleroderma;
- Hypothyroidism.

SYMPTOMS OF XEROPHTHALMIA

- Night blindness;
- Dryness of the eye membrane (conjunctival dryness);
- Corneal dryness;
- Softening of the cornea;
- Itchy, painful, bloodshot eyes.

TREATMENT FOR XEROPHTHALMIA

- Over-the-counter artificial tears;
- A visit wth an eye doctor.

CONCLUSION

This book is written with an emphasis to motivate you **to take responsibility for your own health.** When you take responsibility for your health, you are striving for a healthier lifestyle, which you should try to maintain forever. You will not only enjoy life more, but you will find that your life will be more vibrant, happy, and worth living. Seriously now, just think: you came into this world alone and you will be leaving it alone. Why not choose the way you want to live? We cannot take anything with us when we die, so why not make the best use of all the **resources** we have while we are still alive? Why not make a conscious effort to improve your health? It is not very hard to attain, believe me. If I did it, so can you. The biggest obstacle you will have is your attitude. You will need an attitude adjustment.

Charles R. Swindol states, "Life is 10% what happens to you and 90% how you react to it." Even though you have all the knowledge about how to eat right, you know the importance of exercise, and you're very aware of all the ills of the Western lifestyle and diet, if your attitude towards wellness is not changed, you will not achieve the desired lifestyle change you are anticipating. The pursuit of wellness/good health is a matter of choice. it is the positive attitude you choose to obtain good health, longevity, and happiness. You cannot change your past ways of living (eating, etc.) until you fully realize what they have been doing to your health. You cannot change or escape the fact that big multinational food corporations have been selling food for a profit and not for your health and well-being. You can and should examine and change what you put in your body.

A recent research paper published online in the September 2013 *Journal of the American Heart Association* shows that, even people dealing with heart disease — the number-one killer of adults in this country — will live longer and be stronger, or as we say, live younger if they have a positive outlook and attitude to their health.

Another study that looked at 607 peple in a Denmark hospital found that patients whose moods were overall more positive were 58% more likely to live at least another five years. These people were exercising more, too. The conclusion? "Positive thinking and regular physical activity are really important for life and beauty." This study also brings out a very important fact: "Humour improves immune cell function, helps to ward off illness, decreases your chance of cancer, and apparently also increases your chance of living after heart disease hits." So if you improve on your present lifestyle and incorporate more exercise, proper food, and a stress-management program, do you think your lifestyle will be improved? I do.

Now that we have got the little attitude tune-up out of the way, let us summarize the steps that you need for a brand-new you:

- The importance of the right diet for you. Certain foods will significantly improve your health (Acid-Alkaline Food Guide). Discover if your system is acidic or alkaline and then choose the right type of food/supplement to bring it back to homeostasis. Eat more fresh and organic fruits and vegetables. This new diet is intended to direct you to eat less fats/oils, sugar, cholesterol-rich foods, salt, and alcohol and to consume more whole grains, legumes, fruits, vegetables, and water.
- Be a health-conscious eater. Learn as much as you can about diet. Be well educated nutritionally and commit yourself to eating smartly. Make smart food choices.

- Drink eight glass of purified water daily. Do not drink tap water; it contains chlorine and fluorine. Water flushes and helps to detoxify your body, keeps it hydrated and helps to maintain the pH balance of the bodily fluids.
- Do daily exercise. Walking is the cheapest. The body is designed to walk. Walking helps to alleviate stress and stimulate the lymphatic system. You cannot enjoy optimal health if you are sedentary.
- Incorporate deep-breathing exercises daily.
- Have a spiritual connection with our creator. Remember, we are living on a remarkable planet that he created. Meditate on his greatness and love for us.
- Supplements are important, if you are not eating properly.

In summary, we are an overfed but undernourished people. We are eating too much but we are lacking in the seven key nutrients. We eat too many processed foods that are deficient in nutrients. As a result, a significant portion of our population is chronically deficient of one or more of the essential nutrients.

Please open your minds to change. Remember, you have only one body that cannot be traded in.

GLOSSARY

Acid: a compound that yields hydrogen ions (H+) when in aqueous solution. Acids have a sour taste and turn blue litmus red.

Alkaline: pertaining to substances that increase the relative number of hydroxide ions (OH⁻) in a solution; having a pH greater than 7; basic; opposite of acidic.

Allergen: a type of antigen that produces an abnormally vigourous immune response in which the immune system fights off a perceived threat that would otherwise be harmless to the body.

Allergy: a hypersensitivity disorder of the immune system. Symptoms include red eyes, itchiness, runny nose, eczema, hives, or an asthma attack.

Alopecia: a loss of hair from the head or body.

Alzheimer's: a progressive mental deterioration that can occur in middle or old age due to generalized degeneration of the brain. It is the most common cause of premature senility.

Amino acid: a simple organic compound containing both a carboxyl (—COOH) and an amino (—NH2) group.

Anemia: a condition marked by a deficiency of red blood cells or of hemoglobin in the blood, resulting in pallor and weariness.

Antibiotic: a medicine (such as penicillin or its derivatives) that inhibits the growth of, or destroys, microorganisms.

Antigen: a substance that stimulates the production of an antibody by the immune system. Antigens include toxins, bacteria, foreign blood cells, and cells of transplanted organs.

Biome: the variety of life in the world or in a particular habitat or ecosystem.

Antioxidant: a substance that inhibits oxidation, especially one used to counteract the deterioration of stored food products.

Anxiety: a feeling of worry, nervousness, or unease, typically about an imminent event or something with an uncertain outcome.

Aorta: the main artery of the body, supplying oxygenated blood to the circulatory system. In humans, it passes over the heart from the left ventricle and runs down in front of the backbone.

Artery: a blood vessel that conveys oxygenated blood away from the heart to other parts of the body.

Arthritis: a painful inflammation and stiffness of the joints.

Asthma: a respiratory condition marked by spasms in the bronchi of the lungs, causing difficulty breathing. It usually results from an allergic reaction or other forms of hypersensitivity.

Atom: the smallest unit of an element that retains the chemical properties of the element. Atoms can exist alone or in combination with other atoms forming molecules

ATP: *Adenosine Triphosphate.* The molecule that provides energy for important chemical reactions within a cell.

Autotroph: an organism that is able to form nutritional organic substances from simple, inorganic substances such as carbon dioxide.

Bacteria: a member of a large group of unicellular microorganisms that have cell walls but lack organelles and an organized nucleus, including some that can cause disease.

Base: a compound that yields hydroxide ions (OH-) when in an aqueous solution. Bases have a bitter taste, feel greasy, and turn red litmus blue.

Behaviour: the way in which one acts or conducts oneself, especially toward others.

Biodiversity: the variety of life in the world or in a particular habitat or ecosystem.

Bioflavonoid: any of a group of compounds occurring mainly in citrus fruits and blackcurrants, formerly regarded as vitamins.

Bladder: a membranous sac in humans and other animals, in which urine is collected for excretion.

Blood glucose level: the amount of glucose in the blood. Glucose is a sugar that comes from the foods we eat, and it's also formed and stored inside the body. It's the main source of energy for the cells of our body, and it's carried to each cell through the bloodstream.

Blood pressure: the pressure of the blood in the circulatory system, often measured for diagnosis since it is closely related to the force and rate of the heartbeat and the diameter and elasticity of the arterial walls.

Blood: the red liquid that circulates in the arteries and veins of humans and other vertebrate animals, carrying oxygen to, and carbon dioxide from, the tissues of the body.

BPH: *Benign prostatic hyperplasia* is an enlarged prostate gland. The prostate gland surrounds the urethra, the tube that carries urine from the bladder out of the body.

Brain: an organ of soft nervous tissue contained in the skull of vertebrates, functioning as the coordinating centre of sensation and intellectual and nervous activity.

Cancer: the disease caused by an uncontrolled division of abnormal cells in a part of the body.

Capillary: any of the fine branching blood vessels that form a network between the arterioles and venules

Capsid: the protein coat or shell of a virus particle, surrounding the nucleic acid or nucleoprotein core.

Carbohydrate: any of a large group of organic compounds occurring in foods and living tissues and including sugars, starch, and cellulose. They contain hydrogen and oxygen in the same ratio as water (2:1) and typically can be broken down to release energy in the animal body.

Carbon: the chemical element of atomic number six, a nonmetal that has two main forms (diamond and graphite) and that also occurs in impure form in charcoal, soot, and coal.

Carbonic acid: a very weak acid formed in solution when carbon dioxide dissolves in water.

Carotenoid: any of a class of mainly yellow, orange, or red fat-soluble pigments, including carotene, which give colour to plant parts such as ripe tomatoes and autumn leaves. They are terpenoids based on a structure having the formula C40H56.

Cartilage: firm, whitish, flexible connective tissue found in various forms in the larynx and respiratory tract, in structures such as the external ear, and in the articulating surfaces of joints. It is more widespread in the infant skeleton, being replaced by bone during growth.

Cell membrane: the semipermeable membrane surrounding the cytoplasm of a cell.

Cell: the smallest structural and functional unit of an organism, typically microscopic and consisting of cytoplasm and a nucleus enclosed in a membrane. Microscopic organisms typically consist of a single cell, which is either eukaryotic or prokaryotic.

Chemical reaction: a process that involves rearrangement of the molecular or ionic structure of a substance, as opposed to a change in physical form or a nuclear reaction.

Chemistry: the branch of science that deals with the identification of the substances of which matter is composed; the investigation of their properties and the ways in which they interact, combine, and change; and the use of these processes to form new substances.

Chlorine: the chemical element of atomic number seventeen, a toxic, irritant, pale green gas.

Chlorophyll: a green pigment, present in all green plants and in cyanobacteria, responsible for the absorption of light to provide energy for photosynthesis. Its molecule contains a magnesium atom held in a porphyrin ring.

Cholesterol: a compound of the sterol type found in most body tissues, including the blood and the nerves. Cholesterol and its derivatives are important constituents of cell membranes and precursors of other steroid compounds, but high concentrations in the blood (mainly derived from animal fats in the diet) are thought to promote atherosclerosis.

Chromosomes: a threadlike structure of nucleic acids and protein found in the nucleus of most living cells, carrying genetic information in the form of genes.

Circulatory system: the system that circulates blood and lymph through the body, consisting of the heart, blood vessels, blood, lymph, and the lymphatic vessels and glands.

Colon: the main part of the large intestine, which passes from the cecum to the rectum and absorbs water and electrolytes from food that has remained undigested. Its parts are called the ascending, transverse, descending, and sigmoid colon.

Combustion: rapid chemical combination of a substance with oxygen, involving the production of heat and light.

Compound: a thing that is composed of two or more separate elements; a mixture.

Contraception: the deliberate use of artificial methods or other techniques to prevent pregnancy as a consequence of sexual intercourse. The major forms of artificial contraception are barrier methods, of which the most common is the condom; the contraceptive pill, which contains synthetic sex hormones that prevent ovulation in the female; intrauterine devices, such as the coil, which prevent the fertilized ovum from implanting in the uterus; and male or female sterilization.

COPD: *Chronic obstructive pulmonary disease* (COPD) refers to a group of lung diseases that block airflow and make breathing difficult.

Cytoplasm: the material or protoplasm within a living cell, excluding the nucleus.

Decomposer: an organism, especially a soil bacterium, fungus, or invertebrate that decomposes organic material.

Denaturation: A process in which the folding structure of a protein is altered due to exposure to certain chemical or physical factors (e.g., heat, acid, solvent, etc.), causing the protein to become biologically inactive.

Dendrite: a short-branched extension of a nerve cell, along which impulses received from other cells at synapses are transmitted to the cell body.

Density: the degree of compactness of a substance.

Detoxification: the process of removing toxic substances or qualities.

Diabetes: a metabolic disease in which the body's inability to produce any or enough insulin causes elevated levels of glucose in the blood.

Diet: a special course of food to which one restricts oneself, either to lose weight or for medical reasons.

Digestion: the process of breaking down food by mechanical and enzymatic action in the alimentary canal into substances that can be used by the body.

Disease: a disorder of structure or function in a human, animal, or plant, especially one that produces specific signs or symptoms or that affects a specific location and is not simply a direct result of physical injury.

DNA: deoxyribonucleic acid, a self-replicating material present in nearly all living organisms as the main constituent of chromosomes. It is the carrier of genetic information.

Drug: a medicine or other substance which has a physiological effect when ingested or otherwise introduced into the body.

Duodenum: the first part of the small intestine immediately beyond the stomach, leading to the jejunum.

Ecosystem: a biological community of interacting organisms and their physical environment.

Eczema: a medical condition in which patches of skin become rough and inflamed, with blisters that cause itching and bleeding, sometimes resulting from a reaction to irritation (eczematous dermatitis) but more typically having no obvious external cause.

Electron: a stable subatomic particle with a charge of negative electricity, found in all atoms and acting as the primary carrier of electricity in solids.

Embryo: an unborn or unhatched offspring in the process of development.

Emphysema: a condition in which the air sacs of the lungs are damaged and enlarged, causing breathlessness.

Encephalitis: inflammation of the brain, caused by infection or an allergic reaction.

Endocrine gland: glands of the endocrine system that secrete their products — hormones — directly into the blood rather than through a duct.

Enzyme: a substance produced by a living organism that acts as a catalyst to bring about a specific biochemical reaction.

Epidermis: the outer layer of cells covering an organism, in particular.

Estrogen: any of a group of steroid hormones that promote the development and maintenance of female characteristics of the body. Such hormones are also produced artificially for use in oral contraceptives or to treat menopausal and menstrual disorders.

Eukaryote: an organism consisting of a cell or cells in which the genetic material is DNA in the form of chromosomes contained within a distinct nucleus. Eukaryotes include all living organisms other than the eubacteria and archaebacteria.

Euthanasia: the painless killing of a patient suffering from an incurable and painful disease or in an irreversible coma. The practice is illegal in most countries.

Evolution: the process by which different kinds of living organisms are thought to have developed and diversified from earlier forms during the history of the earth.

Excretion: the process of eliminating or expelling waste matter.

Exon: a segment of a DNA or RNA molecule containing information coding for a protein or peptide sequence.

Exoskeleton: a rigid external covering for the body in some invertebrate animals, especially arthropods, providing both support and protection.

Fat: a natural oily or greasy substance occurring in animal bodies, especially when deposited as a layer under the skin or around certain organs

Fatigue: extreme tiredness, typically resulting from mental or physical exertion or illness.

Fertilization: the action or process of fertilizing an egg, female animal, or plant, involving the fusion of male and female gametes to form a zygote.

Fetus: an unborn offspring of a mammal, in particular an unborn human baby more than eight weeks after conception.

Fibre: dietary material containing substances such as cellulose, lignin, and pectin, which are resistant to the action of digestive enzymes.

Fibromyalgia: a chronic disorder characterized by widespread musculo-skeletal pain, fatigue, and tenderness in localized areas.

Flatulence: the accumulation of gas in the alimentary canal.

Gastric acid: a digestive fluid formed in the stomach. It is composed of hydrochloric acid (HCl) (around 0.5%, or 5000 parts per million) as high as 0.1 M, potassium chloride (KCl) and sodium chloride (NaCl).

Gene: a unit of heredity that is transferred from a parent to offspring and is held to determine some characteristic of the offspring.

Genome: the haploid set of chromosomes in a gamete or microorganism, or in each cell of a multicellular organism.

GERD: *Gastroesophageal reflux disease* is a chronic digestive disease.

Gluten: a substance present in cereal grains, especially wheat, that is responsible for the elastic texture of dough. A mixture of two proteins, it causes illness in people with celiac disease.

Gynecological: the branch of physiology and medicine that deals with the functions and diseases specific to women and girls, especially those affecting the reproductive system.

Heart: a hollow muscular organ that pumps the blood through the circulatory system by rhythmic contraction and dilation. In vertebrates, there may be up to four chambers (as in humans), with two atria and two ventricles.

Herb: any plant with leaves, seeds, or flowers used for flavouring, food, medicine, or perfume.

Heredity: the passing on of physical or mental characteristics genetically from one generation to another.

Heterotroph: an organism deriving its nutritional requirements from complex organic substances

High blood pressure: a common disorder in which blood pressure remains abnormally high (a reading of 140/90 mm Hg or greater).

HIV: *Human Immunodeficiency Virus* is a lentivirus that causes the acquired immunodeficiency syndrome, a condition in humans in which progressive failure of the immune system allows life-threatening opportunistic infections and cancers to thrive.

Homeostasis: the tendency toward a relatively stable equilibrium between interdependent elements, especially as maintained by physiological processes.

Hormone: a regulatory substance produced in an organism and transported in tissue fluids such as blood or sap to stimulate specific cells or tissues into action.

Hydrolysis: the chemical breakdown of a compound due to its reaction with water.

Hygiene: conditions or practices conducive to maintaining health and preventing disease, especially through cleanliness.

Hyperthyroidism: overactivity of the thyroid gland, resulting in a rapid heartbeat and an increased rate of metabolism.

Immune system: a system of biological structures and processes within an organism that protects against disease.

Insulin: a hormone produced in the pancreas by the islets of Langerhans that regulate the amount of glucose in the blood. The lack of insulin causes a form of diabetes.

Intron: a segment of a DNA or RNA molecule that does not code for proteins and interrupts the sequence of genes.

Joule (J): the SI unit of work or energy, equal to the work done by a force of one Newton when its point of application moves one metre.

Joule (J): in the direction of action of the force, equivalent to one 3600th of a watt-hour.

Juvenile Hormone (JH): any of a number of hormones regulating larval development in insects and inhibiting metamorphosis.

Kidney: each of a pair of organs in the abdominal cavity of mammals, birds, and reptiles, excreting urine.

Kinesis: an undirected movement of a cell, organism, or part in response to an external stimulus.

Kinetic energy: energy that a body possesses by virtue of being in motion.

Lactose: a sugar present in milk. It is a disaccharide containing glucose and galactose units.

Ligament: a short band of tough, flexible, fibrous connective tissue that connects two bones or cartilages or holds together a joint.

Lipid: any of a class of organic compounds that are fatty acids or their derivatives and are insoluble in water but soluble in organic material.

Solvents: They include many natural oils, waxes, and steroids.

Lung: each of the pair of organs situated within the rib cage, consisting of elastic sacs with branching passages into which air is drawn, so that oxygen can pass into the blood and carbon dioxide be removed. Lungs are characteristic of vertebrates other than fish, though similar structures are present in some other animal groups.

Lymph: a colourless fluid containing white blood cells that bathes the tissues and drains through the lymphatic system into the bloodstream.

Lymphatic system: the network of vessels through which lymph drains from the tissues into the blood.

Lysosome: an organelle in the cytoplasm of eukaryotic cells containing degradative enzymes enclosed in a membrane.

Meiosis: a type of cell division that results in four daughter cells, each with half the number of chromosomes of the parent cell, as in the production of gametes and plant spores.

Melatonin: a hormone secreted by the pineal gland that inhibits melanin formation and is thought to be concerned with regulating the reproductive cycle.

Meninges: the three membranes (the dura mater, arachnoid, and pia mater) that line the skull and vertebral canal and enclose the brain and spinal cord.

Menopause: the ceasing of menstruation.

Menstrual cycle: the process of ovulation and menstruation in women and other female primates.

Metabolism: the chemical processes that occur within a living organism in order to maintain life.

Mineral: a solid, inorganic substance of natural occurrence.

Mitochondria: *singular* mitochondrion; an organelle found in large numbers in most cells, in which the biochemical processes of respiration and energy production occur. It has a double membrane, the inner layer being folded inward to form layers (cristae).

Mitosis: a type of cell division that results in two daughter cells, each having the same number and kind of chromosomes as the parent nucleus, typical of ordinary tissue growth.

Molecule: a group of atoms bonded together, representing the smallest fundamental unit of a chemical compound that can take part in a chemical reaction.

mRNA: *messenger RNA*; the template for protein synthesis; the form of RNA that carries information from DNA in the nucleus to the ribosome sites of protein synthesis in the cell.

Myosin: a fibrous protein that forms (together with actin) the contractile filaments of muscle cells and is also involved in motion in other types of cells.

Nutrition: the process of providing or obtaining the food necessary for health and growth.

Obesity: the condition of being grossly fat or overweight.

Organ: a part of an organism that is typically self-contained and has a specific vital function, such as the heart or liver in humans.

Osteoporosis: a medical condition in which the bones become brittle and fragile from loss of tissue, typically as a result of hormonal changes, or deficiency of calcium or vitamin D.

Overweight: above a weight considered normal or desirable.

Phytochemical: any of various biologically active compounds found in plants.

Pneumonia: lung inflammation caused by bacterial or viral infection, in which the air sacs fill the lung (*single pneumonia*), or only certain lobes (lobar *pneumonia*).

Pollution: the presence in or introduction into the environment of a substance or thing that has harmful or poisonous effects.

Protein: any of a class of nitrogenous organic compounds that consist of large molecules composed of one or more long chains of amino acids and are an essential part of all living organisms, especially as structural components of body tissues such as muscle, hair, collagen, etc., and as enzymes and antibodies.

Psoriasis: a skin disease marked by red, itchy, scaly patches.

Psychology: the scientific study of the human mind and its functions, especially those affecting behaviour in a given context.

Remedy: a medicine or treatment for a disease or injury.

Reproduction: the natural process among organisms by which new individuals are generated and the species perpetuated.

Respiration: a process in living organisms involving the production of energy, typically with the intake of oxygen and the release of carbon dioxide from the oxidation of complex organic substances.

rRNA: A nucleic acid found in all living cells and play a role in transferring information from DNA to the protein-forming system of the cell.

Stress: a state of mental or emotional strain or tension resulting from adverse or very demanding circumstances.

Sweat: moisture exuded through the pores of the skin, typically in profuse quantities as a reaction to heat, physical exertion, fever, or fear.

Syphilis: a chronic bacterial disease that is contracted chiefly by infection during sexual intercourse, but also congenitally by infection of a developing fetus.

Tear: a drop of clear salty liquid secreted from glands in a person's eye when they cry or when the eye is irritated.

Thorax: the part of the body of a mammal between the neck and the abdomen, including the cavity enclosed by the ribs, breastbone, and dorsal vertebrae, and containing the chief organs of circulation and respiration; the chest.

Urine: a watery, typically yellowish fluid stored in the bladder and discharged through the urethra. It is one of the body's chief means of eliminating excess water and salt and also contains nitrogen compounds such as urea and other waste substances removed from the blood by the kidneys.

UTI: *Urinary Tract Infection* is an infection that affects the part of urinary tract.

Vitamin: any of a group of organic compounds that are essential for normal growth and nutrition and are required in small quantities in the diet because they cannot be synthesized by the body.

Warts: a small, hard, benign growth on the skin, caused by a virus.

Wrinkles: a slight line or fold in something, especially fabric or the skin of the face.

Yeast infection: a fungal infection (mycosis) of any species from the genus candida (one genus of yeasts). Candida albicans is the most common agent of candidiasis in humans.

Zinc: the chemical element of atomic number thirty, a silvery-white metal that is a constituent of brass and is used for coating (galvanizing) iron and steel to protect against corrosion.

REFERENCES

Appleton, Nancy, Ph.D., Heal yourself with natural Foods, New York: Sterling Publishing Co., Inc., 1998.

Balch, James F., M.D. and Stengler, Mark, N.D., Prescription for Natural Cures, New Jersey: John Wiley & Sons, Inc., 2004.

Batmanghelidj, F. WATER for Health, for Healing, for Life, New York: Warner Books, 2003.

Brown, Susan E. & Trivieri, Larry Jr., The Acid Alkaline Food Guide, New York: Square One Publishing, 2006.

Davis, Ben, Rapid Healing Foods, New York: Parker Publishing Company Inc., 1980.

Diehl, Hans, Getting Started, Loma Linda, California: Lifestyle Medicine Institute, 1997.

Diehl, Hans, Reversing Disease with Fork & Knife, Loma Lind CA.: Lifestyle Medicine, 2002.

Edelberg David, Know your Options, Pleasantville, New York: Reader's Digest Association, Inc., 2002.

Holford, Patrick, The Optimum Nutrition Bible, London: 2009

Holmes, Randee, Additive Alert, Toronto, Ontario: McClelland & Stewart, 1994.

Jackson, Adam J., Iridology, Vermilion, London: Random House UK Ltd. 1992.

Libov, Charlotte, Beat Your Risk factors, New York, 1999

William LeGro, High Speed Healing, Pennsylvania: Rodale Press, 1991.

Windridge, Charles, The Fountain of Health, Edinburgh and London: Mainstream Publishing, 1994.

Stengler, Mark, ND, The Natural Physician, Burnaby B.C. Canada: Alive Books, 1997.

Ludington Aileen and Diehl Hans, Take Charge of your Health, Review and Herald Publishing Association, 2001.

Stengler, Mark, ND "The Natural Physician," Alive Books Burnaby, BC Canada, 1997.

Tenney, Louise, Modern Day Plagues, Provo, Utah: Woodlands Books, 1987

Zand, Janet, Allen N. Spreen, James LaValle, "Smart Medicine for healthier Living." New York, Avery Publishing Group, 1999.

INDEX

C

V

W

www.ingramcontent.com/pod-product-compliance
Lightning Source LLC
Chambersburg PA
CBHW062134280526
45788CB00001B/168